Advance Praise for *OMD*

"My top priority in life is to ensure that my children live happy, healthy lives. And I feel an incredible responsibility to teach them the importance of protecting and respecting themselves, others, and the world around them. We now know that incorporating more plant-based foods into our diets is better for overall health . . . and the planet. But it can be difficult to throw together quick, easy, healthful meals that also taste great. In this book Suzy makes it all that much easier, providing all the small things you can do to make a big impact. Filled with wholesome (and super-delicious) recipes, *The OMD Plan* is the solution that every health-minded mama can benefit from."

—*Jessica Alba*

"A timely and empowering guide to take charge of your health—both for your own sake and for the planet's. *The OMD Plan* reveals how one small daily change truly can change our world."

—*Arianna Huffington, founder of HuffPost and founder and CEO of Thrive Global*

"In *The OMD Plan*, Suzy is the perfect guide to gently usher you into plant-based eating. There's simply nothing better you can do for your health, and with *The OMD Plan*'s incremental, nonjudgmental and nutrition-based approach, it's inspiring, achievable—and delicious. Get ready for a health transformation!"

—*Michael Greger, MD*, New York Times *bestselling author of* How Not to Die *and founder of NutritionFacts.org*

"In addition to the well-known nutritional benefits of a plant-based diet, it has now become quite clear that these diets are better for the environment. Suzy Amis Cameron provides clear evidence in support of both of these claims. As well she provides her readers with all manner of tips and tricks to create delicious recipes that will not only be of benefit for their own health, but also that of the natural world. *The OMD Plan* is a book that nourishes our minds as well as providing ways to nourish our bodies."

—*Jane Goodall, PhD, DBE, founder of the Jane Goodall Institute and UN Messenger of Peace*

"The OMD concept really excites me! Anything that nudges us toward making big changes, one step—just one meal—at a time, is a powerful thing. Food interacts with pretty much everything on the planet: our health, the economy, the environment. As Suzy explains, small changes can make a huge difference to our health—and the health of future generations."

—*Jamie Oliver*

"The wave of plant-based eating is making culinary history—and Suzy Amis Cameron shows in *The OMD Plan* that the benefits for your health and the climate are just as groundbreaking. Her book warmly and wisely guides you to make the life-changing shift."

—*Tal Ronnen, founder and chef of Crossroads and* New York Times *bestselling author of* The Conscious Cook

"Cameron's book will appeal to environmentally conscious readers concerned with lifestyle changes that help reduce their carbon footprint."

—*Library Journal*

"Nothing will benefit human health and increase chances for survival of life on Earth as much as the evolution to a vegetarian diet."

–Albert Einstein

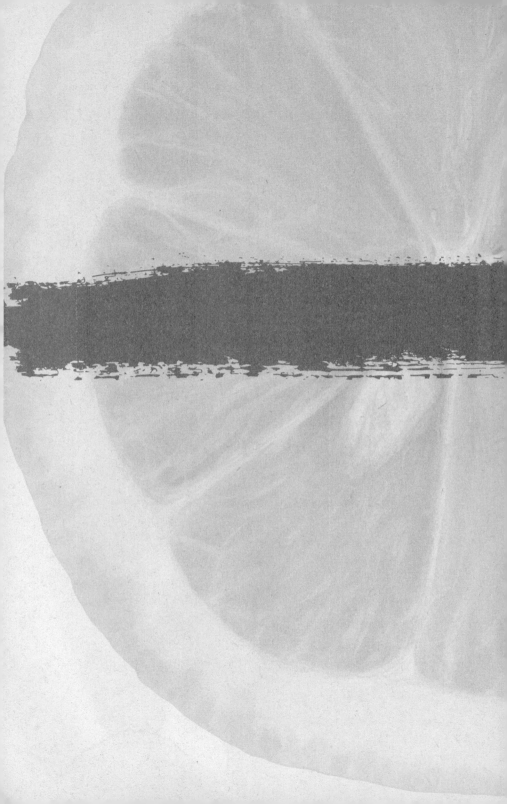

THE

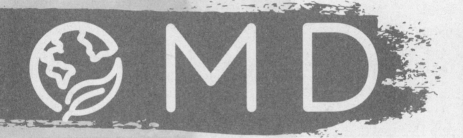

PLAN

PREVIOUSLY PUBLISHED AS *OMD*

SWAP ONE MEAL A DAY TO SAVE YOUR HEALTH AND SAVE THE PLANET

SUZY AMIS CAMERON

WITH MARISKA VAN AALST

FOREWORD BY DR. DEAN ORNISH

ATRIA PAPERBACK

New York • London • Toronto • Sydney • New Delhi

Disclaimer: This publication contains the opinions and ideas of its author. It is intended to provide helpful and informative material on the subjects addressed in the publication. It is sold with the understanding that the author and publisher are not engaged in rendering medical, health, or any other kind of personal professional services in the book. The reader should consult his or her medical, health, or other competent professional before adopting any of the suggestions in this book or drawing inferences from it. The author and publisher specifically disclaim all responsibility for any liability, loss or risk, personal or otherwise, which is incurred as a consequence, directly or indirectly, of the use and application of any of the contents of this book.

ATRIA
PAPERBACK

An Imprint of Simon & Schuster, Inc.
1230 Avenue of the Americas
New York, NY 10020

Copyright © 2018 by Editorial Holding, LLC
OMD flower illustrations courtesy of Angie McArthur

All rights reserved, including the right to reproduce this book or portions thereof in any form whatsoever. For information, address Atria Books Subsidiary Rights Department, 1230 Avenue of the Americas, New York, NY 10020.

First Atria Paperback edition October 2019
Previously published as *OMD*

ATRIA PAPERBACK and colophon are trademarks of Simon & Schuster, Inc.

For information about special discounts for bulk purchases, please contact Simon & Schuster Special Sales at 1-866-506-1949 or business@simonandschuster.com.

The Simon & Schuster Speakers Bureau can bring authors to your live event. For more information or to book an event, contact the Simon & Schuster Speakers Bureau at 1-866-248-3049 or visit our website at www.simonspeakers.com.

Interior design by Tim Shaner, Day&Night Design

Manufactured in the United States of America

10 9 8 7 6 5 4 3 2 1

Library of Congress Cataloging-in-Publication Data

Names: Cameron, Suzy Amis, author. | Aalst, Mariska van, author.
Title: OMD : the simple, plant-based program to save your health, save your waistline, and save the planet / Suzy Amis Cameron with Mariska Van Aalst; foreword by Dean Ornish.
Description: New York : Atria Books, [2018] | Includes bibliographical references and index.
Identifiers: LCCN 2018014225 (print) | LCCN 2018017003 (ebook)
Subjects: LCSH: Veganism—Health aspects. | Nutrition. | Cooking (Natural foods) | Weight loss. | BISAC: HEALTH & FITNESS / Healthy Living. | HEALTH & FITNESS / Weight Loss.
Classification: LCC RM236 (ebook) | LCC RM236 .C26 2018 (print) | DDC 613.2/622—dc23
LC record available at https://lccn.loc.gov/2018014225

ISBN 978-1-5011-8947-0
ISBN 978-1-5011-8948-7 (pbk)
ISBN 978-1-5011-8949-4 (ebook)

For my darling Jim,
In supporting me to fly higher than I ever could have imagined and changing the world together . . .
A Beautiful Journey

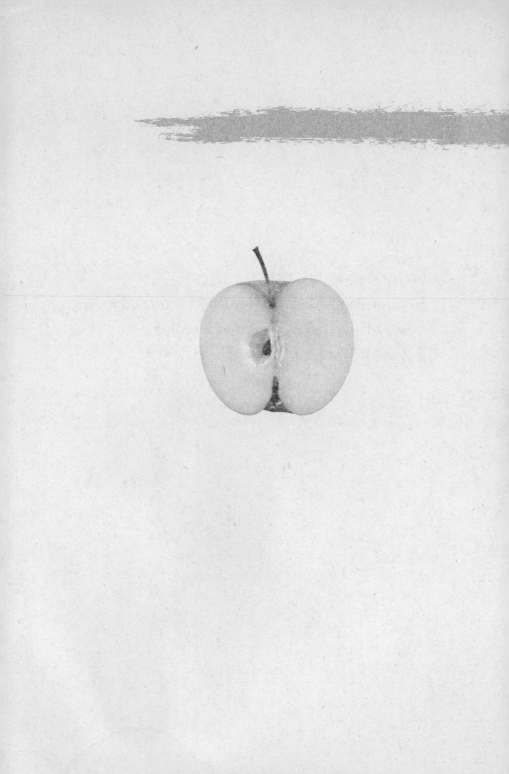

Contents

A Note to the Reader from Rebecca Amis XI

Foreword by Dr. Dean Ornish XIII

Introduction The Simple, Elegant Solution XIX

Part One: Why OMD?

Chapter 1: Our OMD Journey 3

Chapter 2: OMD for Your Health 21

Chapter 3: OMD for the Planet 61

Part Two: The OMD Way

Chapter 4: Prepare to OMD 93

Chapter 5: One Meal a Day 137

Chapter 6: All-In 171

Chapter 7: OMD Recipes 199

Chapter 8: Your Time to Shine 283

Your OMD Resource Well

Calculate Your Own Green Eater Meter Savings 293

Reusable Food Storage and Utensils 294

The OMD Master Pantry List 295

The 14-Day OMD Transition Plan Shopping List 301

The 14-Day All-In Menu Plan Shopping List 305

Converting to Metrics 313

Further Reading, Watching, and Learning 314

Acknowledgments 320

Notes 322

Index 333

A Note to the Reader

Dear Reader,

I am the youngest sibling to my sister Susan—the author of this book. I am a pleasantly content plant-based person and can honestly say this was the way I leaned even as a small child. Being able to whisper sweet nothings into your ear about this book gives me great pleasure!

In the pages ahead, you will hear the story of how OMD—the life-changing program in this book that shows how swapping one dairy- or meat-based meal for a plant-based meal every day can save your health and the planet—came to be. I'm happy to have been a part of that amazing journey, which starts at MUSE School, which I founded with Suzy. It's twelve years old, but it's made great strides in a short amount of time. One of our proudest achievements is that MUSE, the first plant-based school in the nation, has created a legacy of children and families who now know how (and why) to eat one meal a day for the planet!

Easy-peasy, you say? Not!

While going plant-based was not the easiest thing to do at our school, it was the right thing to do. For as Suzy always said, we can't be an environmental school and continue eating and supporting animal agriculture. And I can take it a step further: we can't be a compassionate and emotionally sustainable school and continue to eat animals.

We found that OMD is an ideal way to help students, families, faculty, and staff realize the impact they are making on the environment, their health, and animals' lives. Since implementing the program, we continue to see the benefits that come when we as a school know that we are making an incredible difference. Offering one meal a day for the planet is just that . . . and it's simple! And delicious!

At MUSE, where we have students of all ages, we have found the one meal a day for the planet kinda grows on them. And when it grows on the kid, sometimes the parent catches the bug as well! We are inspiring people to think about education, of course, but also what they eat as it relates to the environment.

And on a personal note, my sister Susan has always been at the helm for all health and environmentally related topics. In other words, sister knows best! I am glad to take this space in the book to share my pride for her. When she sets herself on a mission, there's no stopping her! And now, here's her book, about all things important to her: food and the environment.

So grab some dried kale chips and hummus, curl up with this book, and dig in. You will find her book to be mesmerizing, compelling, and extraordinarily simple!

REBECCA AMIS
Cofounder, MUSE School CA

Foreword

I'm delighted to write the foreword to Suzy Amis Cameron's new book, *The OMD Plan: Swap One Meal a Day to Save Your Health and Save the Planet*. Here's why:

For the past forty years, I have directed a series of randomized controlled trials and demonstration projects proving what a powerful difference comprehensive lifestyle changes can make in our health and well-being—and how quickly this can occur.

These lifestyle changes include a whole-food, plant-based diet naturally low in fat and refined carbohydrates (the one described in *The OMD Plan*); stress-management techniques including meditation and yoga; moderate exercise; and social support (love and intimacy).

In short: Eat well, stress less, move more, love more.

In our research, my colleagues and I used the latest high-tech, state-of-the-art scientific measures to prove the power of these simple, low-tech, and low-cost interventions. We found that these nutrition and lifestyle changes can not only help prevent but often *reverse* the progression of the most common chronic diseases. Our studies have been published in the leading peer-reviewed medical and scientific journals.

I continue to be impressed that the more diseases we study, and the more underlying biological mechanisms we research, the more new reasons and cutting-edge scientific evidence we have to explain why these simple lifestyle changes are so powerful, how transformative and far-ranging their effects can be, and how quickly many people show significant and measurable improvements after implementing them.

We proved, for the first time, that lifestyle changes alone can reverse the progression of even severe coronary heart disease. There was even more reversal after five years than after one year, and 2.5 times fewer cardiac events. We also found that these lifestyle changes can reverse type 2 diabetes and may slow, stop, or even reverse the progression of early stage prostate cancer (and, by extension, early stage breast cancer), high blood pressure, high cholesterol levels, obesity, emotional depression, and early stage dementia.

We found that when you change your lifestyle in these ways, it actually changes your genes—turning on genes that keep you healthy, and turning off genes that promote heart disease, prostate cancer, breast cancer, and diabetes—impacting over five hundred genes in only three months. People often say, "Oh, it's all in my genes, there's not much I can do about it." Knowing that changing lifestyle changes our genes is often very motivating—not to blame, but to empower. Our genes are a predisposition, but they are not our fate.

Telomeres, the ends of our chromosomes that control aging, are like the plastic tips on the ends of your shoelaces—they keep your DNA from unraveling. As we get older, our telomeres tend to shorten, which increases the risk of premature death from a wide variety of chronic diseases ranging from heart disease to cancer to Alzheimer's disease. Our research also showed that these diet and lifestyle changes may lengthen telomeres—and, as your telomeres get longer, your life gets longer. This was the first controlled study showing that any intervention may begin to reverse aging on a cellular level by lengthening telomeres.

Consuming animal protein dramatically increases the risk of premature death independent of fat and carbohydrate consumption. In a study of over six thousand people, those aged fifty to sixty-five who reported eating diets high in animal protein had a 75 percent increase in overall mortality, a 400 percent increase in cancer deaths, and a 500 percent increase in type 2 diabetes during the following eighteen years.

When I began conducting research, I believed that the younger patients with less-severe disease would show the greatest amount of improvement, but I was wrong.

It turned out that the primary determinant of improvements in all of our studies was not how old or sick someone was—rather, it was a direct function of the degree of changes they made in diet and lifestyle. The more they changed, the more they improved in every metric—even telomeres!—that we studied, at any age.

This is a profoundly empowering finding and provides the scientific basis of OMD.

And the more people change their diet and lifestyle, the better they feel, which motivates them to keep doing it. They connect the dots between what they eat and how they feel. ("Oh, when I eat this I feel good; when I eat that, not so well. So I'll eat more of this and less of that.")

This reframes the reason for changing from fear of dying to joy of living. In short, if it feels good, then it's sustainable.

Your brain gets more blood flow, so you think more clearly and creatively, have more energy, need less sleep. You can actually grow so many new brain neurons—a process called neurogenesis—that your brain increases in size in just a few weeks. Especially those parts of your brain that you want to get measurably bigger, such as the hippocampus, which controls memory—as people age, they often start to forget people's names, or where they left their keys. Much of this now appears to be reversible, something that was thought impossible when I went to medical school.

Your skin gets more blood flow, so you may look years younger than your biological age (look at Suzy!). Your heart gets more blood flow, so you have more stamina and can often reverse even severe coronary heart disease. Your sexual organs get more blood flow, so your potency improves.

The biological mechanisms that regulate blood flow—and our health in general—are so much more dynamic than was once thought. The latest research shows that you can get better or worse from eating just one meal, depending on what you consume.

Even a single meal high in animal protein and fat reduces blood flow. For example, Dr. Robert Vogel and his colleagues published a study in the *American Journal of Cardiology* comparing blood flow after a meal high in fat and animal protein (a McDonald's Egg McMuffin, Sausage McMuffin, and two hash brown patties) with a plant-based low-fat meal containing the same number of calories.

After only four hours, blood flow decreased by over 50 percent in those having the McDonald's meal but not in those consuming the plant-based low-fat meal.

When your heart doesn't receive enough blood flow to feed itself, then chest pain (angina) occurs. In our research studies, people with severe heart disease who made the diet and lifestyle changes I recommend reported a 91 percent reduction in the frequency of chest pain after only a few days to a few weeks. Using cardiac PET scans, we measured a 400 percent increase in blood flow to the heart compared to a randomized control group.

This is very meaningful for someone who wasn't able to work, play with their kids, or make love with their partner because of angina and who is now able to do all of these after changing their diet and lifestyle.

And if it's meaningful, then it's sustainable.

I've also learned that if I tell someone, "Eat this, don't eat that," they often want to do just the opposite. Because I've learned that even more than being healthy, most people want to feel in control. This goes back to the first dietary intervention, when God said don't eat the apple—that didn't go very well, and that was God talking.

If you go *on* a diet, sooner or later you're likely to go *off* it—because diets are all about what you can't have and what you must do. And then you may feel shame, guilt, anger, and humiliation, which really are toxic to your health and well-being.

If you're trying to reverse a life-threatening illness such as coronary heart disease, you really do have to make big changes in diet and lifestyle—the pound of cure.

But if you're just trying to feel better, lose a few pounds, or lower your blood pressure, cholesterol, or blood sugar, then you have more latitude—the ounce of prevention.

For most people, what matters most is your *overall* way of eating and living. So if you indulge yourself one day, it doesn't mean you've failed—just eat healthier the next. If you don't have time to exercise or meditate one day, just do a little more the next.

You get the idea.

And what's good for you is also good for our planet. What's personally sustainable is globally sustainable.

As Suzy describes in *The OMD Plan*, to the degree we transition toward a plant-based diet, it not only makes a difference in our own lives, it also makes an important difference in the lives of many others worldwide.

When we realize that something as primal as what we choose to put in our mouths each day makes a difference in the fate of our planet, it empowers us and imbues these choices with meaning.

Again, if it's meaningful, then it's sustainable.

Many people are surprised to learn that eating meat generates more global warming due to greenhouse gases than all forms of transportation combined. In the United States, more than eight billion livestock are maintained, which eat about seven times as much grain as is consumed directly by the entire US population.

It takes about ten times as much energy to eat a meat-based diet as a plant-based diet. Producing 1 kilogram of fresh beef requires about 13 kilograms of grain and 30 kilograms of forage. This much grain and forage requires a total of 43,000 liters of water.

Also, livestock now use 30 percent of the earth's entire land surface, mostly for permanent pasture but also including 33 percent of global arable land to produce feed for them. As forests are cleared to create new pastures for livestock, animal agriculture is a major driver of deforestation: some 70 percent of forests in the Amazon have been turned over to grazing.

So, to the degree we choose to eat a plant-based diet, we free up tremendous amounts of resources that can benefit many others as well as ourselves. We have enough food in the world to feed everyone, if enough people were to eat lower on the food chain. And we can save the planet from melting down.

I find this very inspiring and motivating. When we can act more compassionately, it helps our hearts and our health as well.

As Suzy writes, it's not all or nothing. Start with *one meal a day*. To the degree you move in this direction, there is a corresponding benefit.

You'll look better and feel better, have hotter sex and a cooler planet.

Now *that's* sustainable.

DEAN ORNISH, MD
Founder & President, Preventive Medicine Research Institute
Clinical Professor of Medicine, University of California, San Francisco
www.ornish.com

The Simple, Elegant Solution

This book is a movement and a hopeful call to action. It is also a road map, a Swiss Army knife, and an emotional support system. It has to be all of these things—because that's what most of us need to make the real, sustained changes that save our health and protect our planet. We see the evidence of climate change all around us: wildfires, catastrophic hurricanes, flooding, mudslides. We sense that we've reached a tipping point, that we have to make changes now if we hope to leave a habitable world to our children.

I'm particularly passionate about this because I'm a mom. Like most moms, I have wiped many a tear, runny nose, and dirty bottom. I've been peed on and barfed on, and I would take down anyone who tried to hurt my children. This fierce, mama-bear, protective love is locked into my DNA. It's an instinct, a drive in all moms and dads. All humans! How would we have survived otherwise? Even if we don't have kids, we feel this protective drive about our family, our pets, our friends. This fierce love drives me, every single day, to make the world a better place for all of our children to grow up in.

I'm also a multitasker, like so many of us in this fast world. I have five kids. I'm an entrepreneur, educator, and wrangler of dogs; a former model and actress; and a current daughter, sister, aunt, and mission-driven juggler of way too many things. I've spent many years channeling my fierce protective love into creating initiatives to help save the planet: Red Carpet Green Dress, an organization that challenges and helps the fashion industry to become more environmentally responsible; Plant Power Task Force, an advocacy organization focused on raising awareness and funding highly respected research into the effects of animal agriculture on the environment; MUSE School, an environmental educational organization spanning early childhood to twelfth grade that taps into the passions within each child and awakens their thirst for learning as well as their sense of deep responsibility for protecting the earth and all of its inhabitants, which is also the first plant-based school in the nation (and where OMD first began!); Food Forest Organics, the first completely plant-based market and café in New Zealand; and our newest endeavor, Cameron Family Farms, an exciting chance for us to bring all our philosophies about plant-based eating and environmentalism to life, giving people high-quality, widely available options that will make eating whole-food, plant-based meals more convenient and affordable for all. And for eighteen years, I've been married to an amazing father, husband, and partner, a turbo-charged filmmaker, deep-sea explorer, and Renaissance man, James Cameron. My Jim.

Now, I know my limitations. I'm most definitely *not* a doctor. And I'm not a scientist. Yet I'm a research and information junkie, and I spend a lot of my time trying to get the most credible, up-to-date information out there from real scientists, climatologists, doctors, and researchers. Every ounce of my being that's not devoted to my family is in service to environmental advocacy, caring for our planet, and creating a better, healthier world.

I am fully aware that in so many ways, I've lived a charmed life. I still pinch myself every day, and I know that the big suffering and pain so pervasive in the world isn't often part of my direct experience. Yet I still put my pants on one leg at a time. This year, my father died, my aunt Betsy died, and my mother broke her hip—all in one week. No amount of magic or money in the world can take away grieving and loss.

Along with extreme love and gratitude, I feel a great responsibility to make the world a better place for all our children and many generations to come. In fact, I can barely pass an infant or a kid on the street, or in a grocery store—anywhere—without being reminded of the seriousness and urgency of this commitment.

I WROTE THIS BOOK because I know how hard it can be to get through the day, hurtling from one meeting (or deadline, orthodontist appointment, parent teacher conference, errand, or after-school activity) to another.

I know how many competing demands we have in our lives, each one battling the other for our time, our attention, our energy. Sometimes simply getting through the day feels like a Herculean task.

And whether we're parents or not, we all take care of so many people and problems all the time. Heaping one more consideration onto our shoulders may just be too much. *Oh, great—now I have to take care of the planet too?* Especially when it just seems so huge and unsolvable.

That's the beauty of One Meal a Day for the Planet, or OMD: by switching one meat- or dairy-based meal to one plant-based meal a day, we can slash our personal water and carbon footprint of our diet by about 25 percent. If we go fully plant-based, we can slash it by 60 percent. With this one simple shift, we can cut our risk of heart disease, cancer, and diabetes; lose weight; and even improve our sex lives. With this one shift, we can also help protect the soil, water, and air for all of us. With OMD, we can check off many diverse to-do (or wish-to-do) boxes on our lists simultaneously. We can take care of everyone in our lives—our children, friends, partner, siblings, parents, and especially ourselves—*while* we take care of our community, the planet, and the future, all at the same time.

Talk about the ultimate life-changing hack.

With OMD, I never, ever want to guilt you into changing your behavior. We all know that "guilt" or "should" or "being right" doesn't fuel meaningful and sustained change. My goal is to share how easy, fun, delicious, energizing, and *gratifying* plant-based eating can be. I also want to acknowledge that it can be seriously hard to change the way you're used to eating, shopping, and cooking, so I want to help you gracefully handle the challenges of incorporating more plant-based meals into your life. I'm going to show you dozens of my family's favorite recipes, strategies, and work-arounds that will help you radically boost the nutritional quality of your foods without sacrificing flavor or satisfaction. We'll do this in a way that is at your pace, is to your taste, and fits right into your life, and I promise you'll notice the impact almost immediately. I'm here to testify (occasionally with a bullhorn and pom-pom!) that the transformation can be nothing less than life-changing, and that's my hope for you and for the planet.

That's why we call OMD "the simple, elegant solution." With this one tiny shift, you can:

- 🌏 Lose weight or maintain a healthy weight, easily and effortlessly, without feeling deprived or counting a single calorie
- 🌏 Help reverse fuzzy thinking, low energy, prediabetes, high cholesterol, muscle or joint pain—while you lengthen your life
- 🌏 Become one of those "glowy" people who radiate youth with their clear gorgeous skin, shiny hair, and sparkling eyes
- 🌏 Genetically program your kids for optimal health, setting them up to be lean and strong, with rock-star immunity, for life
- 🌏 Save money once spent on pricey meat and enjoy more nourishing, clean organic produce and delicious sides, sauces, and condiments
- 🌏 Cut down on trips to the doctor, save on medical costs, and, in some cases, reduce or completely eliminate medications

- Eat delicious food that satisfies and surprises you, and wakes up your taste buds to a whole new dimension of exciting foods and flavors
- Enjoy heating up your sex life (while cooling the earth) with increased vitality and newfound energy
- And, oh yeah—*save the planet*

No one wakes up saying, "Hey, I'm going to waste water, pollute our rivers, contribute to climate change."

You may already drive a fuel-efficient (or electric!) vehicle or take the subway or bike or walk to work. Or you may have installed a low-flow showerhead or compact fluorescent lights. Maybe you bring your own shopping bags to the grocery store. You probably recycle—and, shoot, you may even have a compost pile.

You do these things because you care. You want to do your part—you certainly don't want to make matters worse. The truth is, very little we as individuals do comes close to the environmental impact of what we eat. Michael Pollan (the author who coined the phrase, "Eat food. Not too much. Mostly plants") summed it up at the PopTech conference in 2009: "Our meat eating is one of the most important contributors we make to climate change."

It's easy to feel powerless when it comes to climate change. But with OMD, you will realize how much power we *do* have to make things better. I was shocked when I first learned it, but it's true: almost *nothing* you do can help save the earth as much as opting for meat- and dairy-free meals. OMD has been instrumental in helping many people realize and embrace this power, and this book will give you all the tools you need to experience this for yourself.

In part 1, "Why OMD?" I share the story behind OMD, and why it can be such a powerful agent for change, including the surprising research about animal agriculture, how dramatically eating meat impacts Earth's ecosystem, and why opting for even a few more plant-based meals a week makes everyone safer and healthier and the whole world more sustainable. As I said earlier, I'm not a scientist, but I have been very fortunate to work with the best and brightest—when we developed the OMD program at MUSE and while writing this book. Members of the OMD "brain trust"—some of the most respected doctors and researchers in the world—have inspired, advised, and vetted OMD every step of the way.

Then, in part 2, "The OMD Way," I will give you every single stinking idea, trick, tip, tool, suggestion, recipe, strategy—you name it—that I can think of to make OMD as easy, fun, inexpensive, satisfying, and delicious as possible. I'll help you think through exactly how you can implement OMD into your own life, in what ways and at what pace, and help you discover all the different tools you can use to make it happen, like the Green Eater Meter. This metric, developed with Dr. Maximino Alfredo Mejia in the environmental nutrition group of the Department of Public Health, Nutrition and Wellness at Andrews University, quantifies how much of our precious resources—fresh water, fertile land, clean air—we protect when we make these simple swaps for animal products.

The Green Eater Meter will help you visualize and keep track of just how many gallons of water you're saving, how much clean air you're protecting, and even how much natural habitat you're preserving from clear-cutting and deforestation—just from changing one meal a day. Who knew?!

My ultimate goal is to make you fall in love with plant-based eating, so I've also included over fifty delicious OMD recipes that have it all: every possible flavor and texture, every imaginable combination of tastes—sweet, savory, hearty, salty, light, crispy, juicy, smoky. Something for every palate, cooking level, schedule, and budget. Each one of these recipes, contributed by dear family and friends, has its own story.

Because I know people approach change in different ways, I'm offering two plans to choose from. Many prefer to slide in sideways and trick themselves into small changes. If this sounds like your speed, you'll be right at home in chapter 5, "One Meal a Day." Some people do best with an all-in, full-steam-ahead, stand-back-while-I-blow-up-my-kitchen kind of an approach. That's my style, so I definitely have you covered in chapter 6, "All-In."

I've also included some extra tricks to outsmart that knee-jerk rebellious tendency we all can have from time to time, when we *want* to make positive changes in our lives but we just seem to keep tripping ourselves up. (Hello, you anti-authority types. I get you.)

Yet there is one thing *not* permitted on this program: perfection.

We are not about purity; we are all works in progress. Things you will never find here: Shame. Blame. Finger-wagging. "Shoulds." Direct orders.

(Or what our family in Oklahoma loves to say: "Whatcha oughta do.")

No beating yourself up. That's not on the menu!

We recognize that everyone makes decisions about what they put into their mouths on a minute-by-minute, meal-by-meal basis. We know that the secret to honoring your intentions is all about preparation—getting ready, anticipating roadblocks, and creating alternate paths—even if it means your OMD today becomes lunch instead of breakfast, or dinner instead of lunch. (Or you just skip today and start fresh tomorrow.)

Most of all, I want you to recognize that this is not a one-and-done program—this is a lifelong conversation with yourself, your body, your family, your community, your physical world—even your soul. I want to help you develop the tools to honor your own intentions, help you celebrate our sacred role in protecting the earth for future generations, and help you make those healthier, happier choices so simple that they become second nature.

We know that the way any meaningful shift happens is one moment at a time. One choice. One change. One bite. One meal at a time. Let's rewrite our story, together.

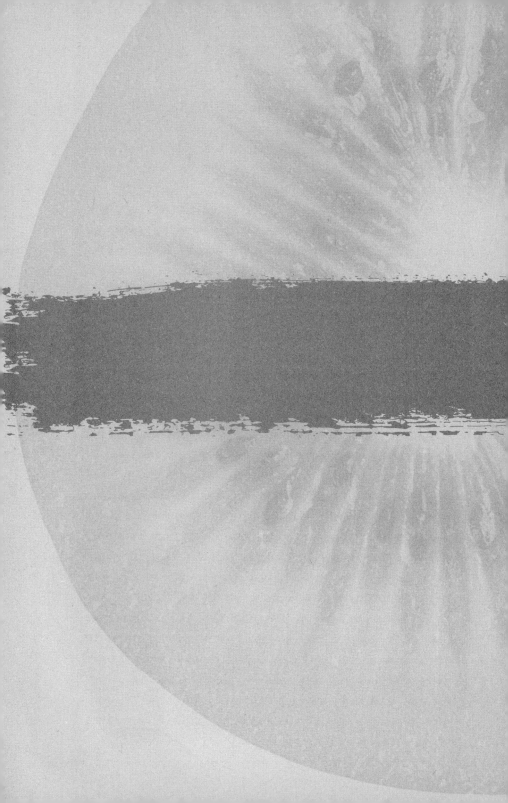

PART ONE

Why OMD?

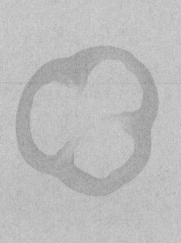

chapter 1

Our OMD Journey

Growing up in Oklahoma, I loved two things: horses and flying. I always planned to be a flying vet. My daddy had taught me how to fly, and I grew up around horses—it seemed the perfect career for me. Spending time on farms, caring for those beautiful, majestic creatures, eating produce straight out of the fields—heaven. I loved that land and those animals fiercely, intently. I wanted to protect them with every bone in my body.

As a teen, all my friends were riding English-style, and I wanted an English saddle for my Western cutting horse from our farm, far from a fancy purebred. But my daddy refused to buy it for me. He said, "I will pay to board and feed Toby, and I'll cover the vet bills, but I am not buying a little bitty saddle." So I started babysitting for fifty cents an hour.

I'd been doing that for a while when my brother got a camera and made me his subject. His pictures turned out good enough, and my aunt Betsy shared my photos with a local modeling agent, Patty Gers. Suddenly I was doing local fashion shows with my big sister, Page, earning in two hours what would've taken me months of babysitting to earn. And when I got the chance to go to New York to meet with Eileen Ford, one of the top modeling agents in the world (thanks again to Aunt Betsy and Patty Gers), I jumped at it.

Well, my first time in New York, over spring break of my junior year, in the span of just four days, I went from sitting in front of Eileen Ford's desk to walking out onto the stage of *The Merv Griffin Show* and being pronounced "The Face of the Eighties" on prime-time television. A totally surreal experience.

Eileen asked me to come back in the summertime to meet with photographers and do interviews. That summer, in a matter of three weeks, I went from standing in Eileen's office to waving goodbye to my parents in Paris, where they left their seventeen-year-old in her new apartment with her newly minted passport.

I quickly learned that the world of high-fashion modeling, which looked so glamorous from the outside, was extremely hard work. Not only did I have to make sure I ate right (to fit in the clothes) and get lots of sleep, I had to show up to work on time, be professional, even navigate international travel.

By the end of the summer, I'd been to Italy three times, to Spain, to London. I had an opportunity to go to Israel and to Morocco. I had also become financially independent.

I started being invited to dinners with interesting, worldly people. I constantly had my nose in a book. I started taking French classes, learning about history, just coming out of my shell. I became a woman in Paris. That experience taught me everything about what a true, authentic education could be when fueled by curiosity and passion.

Claude, my agent, took me around to farmers' markets, taught me the basics of French cooking, and helped me key into the most beautiful aspects of Parisian life. I had always loved vegetables and loved them even more when I was exposed to so many different varieties than just green beans and broccoli. (Although those *haricots verts* were so good!) Well before "nutrient density" became a catchphrase in nutrition, I was learning to eat real food in quantities that kept me in runway shape.

That experience helped protect me from some of the pressures to smoke cigarettes or do drugs or try other "fast" (and dangerous) ways models were using to stay slim. Learning to eat the French way felt healthy and sustainable, gave me a lot of energy—and also taught me even more about the sensory pleasures of vegetables, in all their glorious forms, lessons that would stay with me for life.

By the time I was twenty-one, I'd earned enough to buy my own apartment in New York, in cash—quite an enormous leap from my babysitting wages four years beforehand. At that time, some models were breaking out and becoming actors. My new agency Elite's commercial booker, Davien Littlefield—who would eventually be my manager for sixteen years—kept saying to me, "You should really try acting." Finally, I relented, and she set up my first interview.

That "interview" turned out to be my very first film audition—for a bemused Steven Spielberg. I did my thing, and he kindly smiled and asked, "You don't know anything about this, do you?"

Thankfully, he said there was something "interesting" in my reading, so he introduced me to his protégé, Kevin Reynolds, and that's how I landed my first film, *Fandango*, with Kevin Costner. *Fandango* was also where I met Sam Robards, my first husband. And if I hadn't met Sam, I wouldn't have my eldest son, Jasper.

The Lesson Gets *Real*

I've always been passionate about nature and animals. And I'm one of those lucky people who has been in love with the crunch and the color and the flavors of all kinds of vegetables since I was a kid. Still, I don't think I really understood how it all fit together, on a visceral, spiritual level, until I got pregnant.

After spending four years as a model and then fifteen as an actress, I took the opportunity during my pregnancy with Jasper to relax and eat what I wanted. (I think Jasper was 25 percent crème brûlée.) I gained fifty pounds, and I loved every delicious ounce.

Being pregnant is a perfect window for paying attention to what your body is telling you. You're more attuned to what your skin is telling you, what your energy level is telling you. You start to realize that when you're pregnant and you're full, you're *full*. There's no way around it; there's no more room.

I can remember one night riding in the car with a big Pyrex measuring cup, drinking my precisely measured two cups of milk as prescribed by the *What to Expect When You're Expecting* ladies— had to get that milk quota in! I was also eating a lot of veggies and learning all about organic food. All along, I had this focus on protein—I was constantly being bombarded with messages that I needed to eat meat and drink milk to be strong and grow a strong healthy baby. (I wish I had a dollar for every time my mother had said to us, "Now, you girls remember to drink your milk.")

Then, once Jasper was born, an even deeper, instinctive protective mechanism kicked in. Everything that my little baby ate, touched, sat on, or slept in had to be as pure as possible. I became hyperfocused on potential toxins in the environment. When Jasper was about eighteen months old and Sam was working in New York, I started doing two movies, one in Chicago and one in South Carolina. My sister Rebecca was a lifesaver—she was Jasper's nanny and my "wife" rolled into one. I would come home from a long day of filming, and she would have dinner ready for us—tons of vegetables, soups, salads, rice cakes—this whole big spread. I must've really loved it because I've eaten that way ever since. It's funny to think back on that now—there was a time many years ago when I was eating very close to plant-based, without putting a label on it, and I remember feeling great.

Sam and I split up when Jasper was three.

Then, when Jasper was six, I met Jim.

Cleaning Out the Cupboards

Jim and I started out on opposite ends of the food spectrum. We first met when he cast me in *Titanic*, and we started dating after I wrapped my part in the film. When I went to his house, I would stand in front of his pantry and stare at the cans of meat chili and sardines, and say to myself, "There is not one thing I can bring myself to eat here." Literally the only thing I could find to eat was Rice Krispies.

Once we were married, I slowly shifted the composition to an organic pantry—I added some things, replaced some things. As each of our three children were born, I started moving some of the less healthy stuff up to the higher shelves. We carried on living our busy lives—Jim making his films, me opening MUSE School with my sister, together raising our kids.

Then one day, about a decade after we first got together, Jim came in and looked in the pantry and said, "This pantry is full and there is not one thing in here that I want to eat." He was joking, of course. But I think a moment like this comes in most marriages or cohabitations—when what feels right and tastes good to one person might be exactly the opposite of what the other person craves or needs to feel nourished. Making changes as a family takes a lot of diplomacy, patience, and understanding. Yet those changes in the pantry were just the warm-up for the big one we were about to make, together.

In the spring of 2012, I thought we were doing really well on the food front—our family ate organic grass-fed beef, free-range chicken, omega-3-packed eggs, in addition to a ton of vegetables. We had organic milk and cheese and yogurt. We grew most of our own produce and had goats at our ranch (and made yogurt and cheese from their milk). We were operating under the assumption that we needed that milk, we needed that meat, we needed those eggs. And we were feeding everyone at MUSE the same way. The protein! We had to have our meat and dairy!

At the same time, I had just turned fifty, Jim was heading toward sixty, and we were also starting to see some of our siblings and friends develop health concerns. I began looking at Jim and myself and wondering if we were next. We both have heart disease and cancer in our families. I didn't want that for us. I knew there had to be another way—but what?

One day, I was headed to our workout room, and I picked up the DVD of the documentary *Forks Over Knives*. It had been on my shelf for nine months. My friend Elliot Washor had recommended it to me, and he kept talking about it for over a year. So that day, May 6, 2012, I grabbed it, thinking, "OK, fine, I'll watch this today."

Well, fast-forward to ten minutes later—and I had to get off the treadmill and just sit down and watch the film. It felt like my entire world was falling apart. Here I thought I was giving my family and the children at MUSE the best and highest quality of foods. But now I felt bamboozled. I felt betrayed.

Forks Over Knives is a documentary based on the works of Dr. T. Colin Campbell, a nutritional biochemist from Cornell University, and Dr. Caldwell Esselstyn, a former surgeon from the Cleveland Clinic. The movie traces the experiences of a group of people who used plant-based eating to reverse degenerative disease. Watching that film, I felt like I had been lied to my whole life; that the people and institutions I'd trusted to take care of us had been misleading us for generations, pushing aside the health and well-being of children and families. I heard the echoes of all those nutritional maxims I'd taken on faith: *You need meat to build muscle. You need milk to build strong bones and teeth.* And now I knew it was a gigantic, decades-long, lobbyist-supported lie for the meat and dairy industries' bottom line.

Shaken to my core, I only knew that I had to have Jim watch with me. I had to know if the film would affect him the way it had affected me. I dearly hoped it would, because I already knew my life had been irrevocably changed.

The very next day, I sat there and watched him as he watched it, but he didn't say a word. The second the film ended, he stood right up, walked out of the room, and by the time we got to the kitchen, he said, "We can't have any animal products in our house anymore."

Twenty-four hours later, we had cleared everything out. Bam!

Now, that's just how Jim and I roll—we commit to something, and we go all in. No turning back.

In the following months, we gobbled up as much info as we could about plant-based eating. I found out that part of that gorgeous glow people always talk about comes from the fact that plant-based eaters literally age more slowly, on a cellular level, than meat-and-dairy eaters. Plant-based eating increases the body's own antiaging activity by raising our level of telomerase, the enzyme that makes it possible for our genes to repair themselves, and plant-based bodies have less inflammation, the process that drives cellular aging and can make us look (and feel) old before our time. For every extra 3 percent of plant protein we eat, we cut our risk of death by 10 percent.[1] And I read studies showing that compared to people whose diets are meat- and dairy-focused, people who focus their eating on fruits, vegetables, nuts and seeds, and whole grains:

 Live on average almost 3.6 years longer[2]
 Have a 24 percent lower risk of developing heart disease[3]
Have a 25 percent lower risk of developing diabetes[4]
Have a 43 percent lower risk of developing cancer[5]
Have a 57 percent lower risk of developing Alzheimer's disease or dementia[6]

And now here we are, over six years later, and we're both healthier than we've ever been. Almost no illness. Jim lost thirty-plus pounds. He can work out harder and longer than ever, run for miles barefoot on the beach, do yoga twice a week. He kickboxes. On Mondays and Thursdays he works out for three hours, then takes two- to three-mile walks with me at night—can't slow this guy down. He has seemingly aged in reverse.

My diet hasn't changed that dramatically—I always was a sucker for salads and soups, those foods I learned to love in Oklahoma, in my days in Paris, and with my sister. Now that I'm 100 percent plant-based, I find that I can work out harder than ever. My recovery is better than ever. I can easily slide into any pair of pants in my closet, without a second thought, without ever monitoring what I'm eating or how much. No more fifteen-pound fluctuations. I am in better shape now than I was in my twenties.

Now, did I initially have cravings for yogurt and cheese? Yeah. (Wait, let's get real: I was totally addicted to yogurt and cheese.) After living in Paris, I know a good cheese when I see it (or smell it). Have I ever craved a nice creamy cup of black tea with half-and-half and vanilla on Christmas morning? You bet. But those cravings have become more and more rare as the years go on, as my tastes have changed and the plant-based marketplace has exploded with satisfying, super-yummy alternatives.

On the whole, I've been resolute, as has Jim—and certain things made the transition easier for us. First, we are lucky to have each other as partners. We can support each other because we share this mission, a love for the environment and a feeling of responsibility to do all we can; plant-based eating has become our common project. And this shift was made possible by that moment with *Forks Over Knives*, seeing how we'd been lied to by the meat and medical industries, and wanting to reclaim our health after that sense of betrayal. It's kind of like the feeling you'd get when you binged on a certain food as a kid, then got sick from it—you just can't see the appeal anymore. All you can see is how bad it makes you feel.

Healthier for Us, Healthier for the Earth

Like many couples, our walks and time alone are essential, a non-negotiable that we've scheduled since the early days of our relationship. With a dog and a stick to throw, we set off to reconnect and work through the minutiae of raising kids, work, and marriage. We talk about the health of our parents, the puppy that's waking me up all night, our five kids, a new person we've met; we wrestle with challenges and share new ideas and projects. It's sacred composting. We both have big lives, big families, and big purpose. By handling the domestic stuff and getting it out of the way, we can get to the heartbeat of our life together.

A few months after our shift to plant-based eating, Jim and I were up at our ranch for summer break. Jim was writing the *Avatar* sequels. I was doing the summer hustle with our three-of-five kids still at home and various cousins and friends and dogs. Jim had started to share all he knew about the environmental impact of animal agriculture, pointing me to dozens of books and documentaries. Again, I was gutted. I learned that animal agriculture was responsible for the loss of 70 to 80 percent of the Amazon rain forest. That 17 percent of all global fresh water usage went to livestock production. That animal agriculture is one of the leading causes of extinction. And dead zones in the ocean. And deforestation. And the final gut punch? That animal agriculture contributes 14.5 percent of all human-caused greenhouse gas emissions, *more than the entire transportation sector combined.*

When I'd learned about the health effects of animal products, I'd been knocked for such a loop. Now I was stunned again. "You're kidding—not only is this way of eating killing us, but it's also polluting the planet? Animal agriculture and our overwhelming appetite for meat and dairy are *creating* climate change?"

Walking on the beach near the ranch, we talked about how to get our family and friends interested in plant-based eating and how to expand the circle. We started thinking about environmental impacts: If each of those people could eat more plant-based meals, how much would the environmental savings multiply with more and more of us eating sustainably? We started getting excited.

Now, let me add, parenthetically, what may be obvious to anyone who's seen Jim's movies: My husband is a doomsday kind of guy. (I mean, *Aliens*? *The Terminator*? *Avatar*?) He has a T-shirt with a bottom line that reads, "Hope is not a strategy." He's emergency-ready and primed for disaster. We'd been talking about climate change for a long time. The prospect of the apocalypse of climate change had always been easier for him to imagine than for me. For *years*, I would come home from depressing environmental NGO meetings, where we'd been regaled with slide after slide of environmental degradation, and I would be so disheartened that I instinctively shifted into being the cheerleader. "It'll be OK! We're going to clean up the oceans! We'll recycle, change our light bulbs, drive a Prius. . . ."

When he used to listen to my chirpy, upbeat ideas for saving the planet, he'd smile kindly and say, "That's great, babe—but it's not going to move the needle." He was over there thinking big system change, realizing that those incremental changes, even when adopted broadly, would never make up the difference necessary.

But that night on the beach, Jim turned to me. "For the first time in my life, I have hope," he said. "The more people we can get to go plant-based, the better chance we'll have of addressing climate change. Doing that *will* move the needle."

I stopped. Had I just heard the man use the word *HOPE*?! The man who had imprinted aliens launching out of stomachs and Arnold Schwarzenegger going postal on our cultural memory?

Jim's words galvanized me, lighting a fire that's since become an inferno.

We can do this.

Going plant-based changed everything. We started to realize that every meal *did* matter—that even small steps toward plant-based eating can have a tremendous impact on the environment, and that we could start to have a massive impact *right now*, at our own kitchen tables. We don't need a single elected official to do a single noble thing; we don't have to wait for the politicians to lead. *We* have to lead, and politicians will follow.

Remember those Viking ships of yore, with those long oars? The more rowers a ship had, the faster it would go. I keep thinking we are all on a boat like that—the more people who get on the boat, the more arms we'll have, rowing in the same direction, and the faster it will go.

As I tell more and more people about plant-based eating, I've imagined more and more people getting on our trusty Viking ship. I've been overjoyed to see how fast the message has spread, how many lives have been changed, and how great of an impact we can have every single day.

We can commit this revolutionary act right now. We can all jump on board together, all start rowing in the same direction. We can get where we want to be—*fast*. All we have to do is change our lunch order.

And, funnily enough, that's how the OMD concept started: with lunch.

The Birth of OMD

The idea of eating One Meal a Day for the Planet was born at MUSE School, the passion- and interest-based learning environmental school based in Calabasas, California, that I founded with my sister Rebecca Amis. We poured our souls into creating MUSE. When we started almost thirteen years ago, we wanted to create an innovative, energizing learning environment for our own kids—and then we quickly realized that we wanted to share that kind of experience with many others.

When my kids first started school, I was terrified. I thought back to my own school experiences—how I'd dreaded school as a child, how I had focused so much on fitting in. I watched our older children, Jasper and Josa, suffer in demoralizing, stifling, punitive school settings. Rebecca's kids were similar in age to mine, and she has a master's in early childhood education. In Wichita, Kansas, she'd opened a Reggio Emilia early childhood program, a child-centered program that utilizes self-directed, experiential learning in relationship-driven environments. When she introduced me to this method of teaching, I was sold. We believed in this approach to our core, and we decided to go for it.

We began MUSE with the belief that true learning is possible when children are permitted to engage in their passions. We articulated a mission, inspiring and preparing young people to live consciously with themselves, one another, and the planet, with a focus on a sustainable campus.

We believed in the mission with all our hearts, and pursued it in every way possible—we *thought*. Yet a few years into being plant-based at home, and after working very hard to try to fulfill our vision of a carbon-neutral, energy-independent campus, Rebecca and I realized we weren't honoring *our* own hearts. Rebecca, her husband, Jeff, Jim, and I had already had a major awakening in the food we ate, and we'd all gone plant-based. We were sharing it with everyone in our lives—we had our own little community, trading notes and recipes. But Rebecca and I hadn't yet translated it to the school. We knew we needed to go 100 percent plant-based to truly model a 100 percent sustainable and environmentally focused school. And while we'd always thought we were serving these kids the best possible food, we now realized we were unintentionally poisoning them. And the planet.

We assumed everyone would feel the same. So, in January 2014, we joyfully scheduled a screening of the documentary *Forks Over Knives* during a professional development day and told the teachers and staff of our plans: We were going to take eighteen months to transition, and by September 2015, we would be a fully plant-based school. The first plant-based school in the nation.

Weren't they excited?

Well, suffice it to say . . . not exactly. We encountered more resistance than we had anticipated, to put it mildly. About one-third of the staff just sat there with their arms crossed—I could almost see their heels digging in. They didn't even want to watch the film—they thought we'd be showing them videos about baby cows being led to slaughter. (Spoiler: No baby cow slaughter.)

One staffer, let's call her Ellen, was adamantly opposed. Wasn't having any of it. Didn't even want to watch the video. But she did—with arms crossed the whole time.

Well, that was in the spring, before summer break. Fast-forward three months, and by fall, Ellen was back—hair gleaming, eyes shining. Arthritis gone. Energy through the roof. Finally able to sit on the floor with her kids again and move around easily. Complete one-eighty from the spring. It was such a beautiful sight to see her so happy and energetic, just glowing.

Why, Ellen, you little sneak. After kicking up such a fuss, she had gone home over the summer and tried it—she went plant-based. She lost thirty pounds and completely transformed her life in a matter of months.

Thereafter, we saw this same transition happen among staff members again and again. The assistant head of school, same thing—forty pounds gone, ditched his medications. Literally had to buy a whole new wardrobe. PR manager, thirty pounds. Given a clean bill of health after some tricky thyroid issues.

With those initial skeptics now fully on board, it was time to float the idea with the parents.

Again, the same reaction: *No. Way.*

So many people were good and kind, devoted to the planet,

committed to the mission of the school . . . and extremely disappointed in us. Let's be frank: it was full-on mutiny.

People were up in arms. *How will my child get enough protein? Why is he eating so much rice? He can't make it through the day without his beef jerky!*

I recognized their resistance—hadn't I been there myself? Both Jim and I had been convinced animal-based protein was essential to health, too, so I could understand their reluctance. The pro-meat messages we've all received for so long are lodged deep into our collective belief system around food. We all need a little deprogramming from a lifetime of misinformation.

My sister and I remained resolute—we needed to find a way. We worked with the parents—we listened to all their concerns, we talked everything through with Kayla, our brilliant chef. We experimented and we tinkered and we talked some more. We created MUSE Talks: Once a month, plant-based experts from all different disciplines came in to spend the whole day with our school community. They'd talk to the kids—from the little bitty ones all the way up to the high schoolers, in developmentally appropriate ways. Rip Esselstyn, former triathlete and author of *The Engine 2 Diet*, along with Rich Roll, ultra-endurance athlete and author of *Finding Ultra*, talked to them about being strong and healthy and working out. Dr. Neal Barnard, founder of the Physicians Committee for Responsible Medicine and author of seventeen books, talked to them about protecting their health with plant-based eating. *Veganist* author Kathy Freston and performing artist/ animal activist Moby talked to them about animals. Celebrity vegan chef Tal Ronnen did a beautiful and super-yummy cooking demonstration for us. And then we'd do a nighttime presentation to the parents and the general public. We served plant-based meals and a glass of wine, and everyone learned from an amazing roster of brilliant people. All these dynamic, plant-based advocates taught us an enormous amount about plant-based eating and how to move toward it in a fun, easy, and satisfying way.

During these discussions, I'll admit it—I was in heaven. I'll never forget when T. Colin Campbell came to meet with us—there he was, the groundbreaking author of *The China Study*, the paradigm-shifting book that helped inspire the creation of *Forks Over Knives*, right there in the driveway. I was star-struck; I don't get star-struck normally, but he is a superstar to us. Same thing happened when I talked to Dr. Michael Greger, author of *How Not to Die*, a bestselling book on plant-based lifestyle (and a highly entertaining video star on his impeccably researched website, NutritionFacts.org), on the phone. I was so nervous. I felt like a giddy groupie, I was so excited to talk to him!

This roster of geniuses supported us through the transition and has developed into a giant, committed OMD brain trust that has continued to collaborate with us on everything from those first OMD menu plans to information nights and ongoing curriculum to developing products and programs, and even to helping inform public policy and international advocacy campaigns. We are so lucky to partner with these passionate visionaries as we all work hard to spread the word and create more plant-based solutions for public health and climate change.

Throughout that entire eighteen-month OMD transition process, the goal of many of these inspiring talks was simply to reassure parents that it would be okay: "It's just one meal. It's just one meal a day." After all, we were only talking about lunch here—everyone was welcome to eat as they wished at home.

Still, many heels remained dug in. The school community seemed stuck.

Part of me just wanted to say, "Fine. You can feed them eggs and bacon in the morning and a big burger at night."

Then one day, Rebecca's husband, Jeff King, who is the head of school, just said, "OMG, people. It's just OMD."

And OMD: One Meal a Day for the Planet, was born.

All of a sudden, the light bulb went off: People really understood. And opened up. They saw that we weren't asking them to become vegan, or even vegetarian. We were just talking about lunch and snacks. We were just saying, "In this one place, at this one time each day, we are going to make a conscious choice not to use animal products and dedicate that meal to healing the earth."

Finally, we did it. We won hearts and minds. And OMD became the motto of the MUSE lunchroom.

The results of the whole process were truly amazing. We found a way to get everyone what they needed. The parents were reassured by doctors and nutritionists that their children's protein and other nutritional needs were being met. The kids were reassured that they weren't going to be eating hay bales every day. The staff were reassured that the kids' plant-based lunches would sustain them through their afternoons of outdoor exploration and passion projects. The students really threw themselves into growing their own food in our campus gardens. They've increased their yield to the point where now, MUSE students tend 150 raised beds and grow 80 to 90 percent of the produce they eat in the lunchroom every day.

We have conversion experiences with kids all the time. They start school saying, "I hate eating anything green." The next thing you know, a month in, they're eating sautéed green beans sprinkled with flaxseed oil. It helps that the kids are in the garden growing the beans themselves, so they're able to taste them right off the vine.

We have kids cutting down on their allergy medication. Kids who'd been less active now dropping pounds and climbing hills. Kids who'd been on medication for ADD and ADHD and ABCDEFG now feeling calmer and more focused, even able to get off their meds completely.

These days, rather than resistance and pushback, we have families who seek us out *because* we are plant-based. Families want to have their children on a dye-free, toxin-free, pesticide-free campus, and they want to know where the food their children are eating is coming from. We even had two families move all the way from New York to have their children attend MUSE.

These days, every school year begins with an invitation for students to join together in the OMD mission and to sign their names to a pledge: *I want to make this happen. Together with my school community, I will eat One Meal a Day for the Planet, or Two, or All-In.* We celebrate this moment with them, and the children have *embraced it*, on a soul level—they've made the connection between what they put on their plate and the air they breathe and the water they drink and the future of their planet. They've internalized this connection, in part, by following this simple practice that allows them to *live it*, every single day.

Together, We Can Heal the World

I have learned a tremendous amount during this process. In talking to my family, the teaching staff, the students, and their families, I've learned so many different concerns that people have when making this transition: all the fears, the misconceptions, the cravings. And through trial and error, I've learned how to craft an approach that can satisfy even the most reluctant kid (or adult) and lure them into embracing OMD as their own.

I've seen the seemingly miraculous transformations that have come about from this one small change—the health benefits never cease to amaze me. (I call these "benefit effects"—in contrast to the damaging "side effects" we get from eating the standard meat-based diet.) And I know that these changes are making a measurable impact on our precious Earth, helping to keep her air, waters, and soil clean for future generations. I know without a doubt that if everyone changed just one meal a day, we could start to reverse our course to save our planet. Just one person and one meal can have that much impact.

That's my inspiration for sharing OMD with you. And I want you to succeed, which is why I've designed this book as an all-in-one resource to help you transition to this new way of eating. First I'll share findings from the large and growing body of research proving plant-based nutrition can help reverse a variety of chronic diseases, including diabetes and heart disease, and reduce your risk of cancer. You'll hear stories from people who've used OMD to shift toward more plant-based eating, and how it helped them lose weight, feel more energetic, and even think more clearly. You'll learn why each meal you eat has such a tremendous impact on the environment. Then I'll share everything you need to get ready for OMD, including dozens of tips, tools, and techniques to help you troubleshoot the rough spots so you can discover how delicious and easy it can be to eat more plants. And finally, you can explore over fifty beloved, simple, satisfying recipes from MUSE and my family and friends, each one tried and tested in real family kitchens and approved by even the most resistant carnivores.

I promise you that within a short period of eating more plant-based meals, you'll feel stronger, sharper, and more energetic than you have in years—perhaps healthier than you ever have. And you'll feel even better knowing that you're doing everything within your power to help heal the planet. (Because, boy, does she need our help!)

Now, you and I don't live together, so I'm not going to be able to sit down with you for an hour and a half so we can watch *Forks Over Knives*—so I'm going to pull in some help. Next you'll hear from our OMD medical brain trust as they share decades of compelling research that has powered millions of plant-based health makeovers. My goal is to show you exactly what the OMD way of eating can do for the health of your entire family, not just now, or in twenty years, but for generations and generations into the future.

chapter 2

OMD for Your Health

My dear friend and former manager, Davien, tells this great story of her transition to whole-food, plant-based eating. She'd been carrying some extra pounds for a while and had a health scare that normally comes when people are a little bit older. "On the very same day, I received your gift of a bag of books about plant-based eating, and a freezer box full of steaks from a rancher in Oklahoma," she laughs. "Has there ever been a clearer moment of truth?" Two messengers, both from Oklahoma, on the very same day.

Davien thought, *OK, I've already eaten more steak than most people will consume in a lifetime. The path forward for me is to get rid of those elements in my life.* She gave the steaks to friends in her neighborhood in New York, and started the next day on her course as a plant-based eater. Since then, she hasn't looked back—she's been a self-proclaimed "happy vegan" for over five years. She's also lost sixty pounds over that time, bit by bit. "I've carried a lot of weight my whole life," she says. "When you gain weight, acquiring it is a slow process. And the same is true when you lose weight by going vegan.

"I don't think about myself as being on a diet," she says. "Weight loss just happens to coexist with the plant-based choices that I make." She feels a lightness and clarity, and her arthritis symptoms have basically disappeared.

Davien is one of my best (and most beloved) examples of the positive, happy, healthy changes that come after the plant-based epiphany—but I have heard hundreds of these types of stories. People who were given terminal prognoses, changed their diet, and have been in remission for a decade-plus. People who've reversed their heart disease and diabetes, gotten off all their medications. People whose symptoms of allergies, arthritis, even autoimmune conditions like MS have been radically reduced, just from eating plant-based. I'll share some of the overwhelming proof that eating the OMD way—with more plant-based foods and fewer animal products—could truly be a silver bullet for many of our country's most dangerous chronic health conditions. We'll also talk about how whole-food, plant-based nutrition can help parents set their kids up for their strongest, healthiest, longest lives—and pass along those strong genetic benefits for generations. I hope you come away from this discussion understanding the enormous power in plant-based foods, and how doing OMD together can be a gateway into a whole new level of health for you and your entire family.

A Habit We Can Break

Most people I know grew up with meat right in the center of their plate—and we didn't even question it. Think of "meat and potatoes"—it's a universal metaphor for something basic, central, fundamental. A given. For years, we have been sold on the health value of meat and encouraged to believe that meat is the proper foundation of a meal.

Then add on all the cultural and familial traditions, social bonding, personal identity, religious observance: your grandmother's spaghetti sauce, your father's chicken soup, the Thanksgiving turkey. All these emotional associations go into our meals and are at least as important as the actual physical ingredients. For generations, meat has been sold not only as a medically healthy and necessary food, but as an emotionally healthy one as well. Real men eat meat, the redder, the better. Meat keeps your growing children happy and healthy. Meat brings everyone together around the table. Beef. It's what's for dinner.

The message was clear: meat is good for our bodies and good for our souls.

But nothing could be further from the truth. What happens when you actually look at the medical research and data? Do meat and other animal products improve your health? Do vegan diets sap your strength?

Well, *Forks Over Knives* forever changed the way I looked at that—I realized that our bodies are stronger and more resilient when we *don't* eat meat than when we do. And many believe we were never even meant to eat meat at all. "Many people imagine that human beings are naturally meat eaters, as if we're somehow honorary dogs and cats," says Dr. Neal Barnard, a member of the OMD brain trust, adjunct associate professor of medicine at the George Washington University School of Medicine and Health Sciences in Washington, DC. "But look in your cat's mouth: long saber teeth. Then look in the mirror at your own: canines no longer than your incisors. That change occurred at least three and a half million years ago."

Dr. Barnard believes we are naturally herbivores, and only started to behave as carnivores during the Stone Age, when we developed stone tools and hatchets and arrowheads that allowed us to kill and eat animals we otherwise couldn't have. Now we have an entire industry dedicated to providing steady doses of meat every day. But that is not our natural diet, says Barnard.

Our intestines also look nowhere near what a pure carnivore's look like. Carnivores have short intestines, about three times the length of their bodies, to speed meat through the body quickly so pestilent bacteria or microbes have less of a chance of being absorbed. In contrast, the digestive systems of ruminant herbivores, like cows, are about thirty times the length of their bodies. That's a big reason why they need to eat all day long, to keep themselves constantly fed while they're digesting. (And, as we'll talk about in chapter 3, that keeps them burping all that methane, as well.)

Some say that we humans should really be considered "frugivores"—we have a completely different system than true carnivores or herbivores. The combination of various enzymes and the sheer distance of our thirty-foot-long intestinal tracts allows us to mash up and extract every single nutrient possible from the food we eat. When we eat plant-based foods, our bodies digest them within a day. (One might say, like clockwork.) If we're eating meat, though, the process is slowed way down, taking at least two days, sometimes even longer. And that means our bodies have that much more time to extract all the microbes, viruses, bacteria, heavy metals, persistent pesticides, and other environmental toxins that animal has consumed (and concentrated in its meat) during its lifetime too. Not so good.

YOUR OMD BIO-GOALS

As you read this chapter, try to take honest stock of your own health situation, that of your family, and what goals you might have.

1. **What cards were you dealt?** Using a family tree template, try to capture as much information about your family's health history as possible. Do you see any common threads? Perhaps heart disease, cancer, dementia? Autoimmune conditions? Note everything down so you can get the full picture.

2. **How did your family play those cards?** Next to each person, jot some quick notes about their general level of self-care:

Were they an athlete? A couch potato? A smoker? Did they take vitamins, wear sunscreen, go to the doctor? Try to capture as much information as you can remember.

3. *How does your current branch look?* Now, repeat the process for you and your immediate family: Have any issues already come up? How have you been addressing them? How might you be complicating your health picture?

4. *How would you like your future to look?* Take out a fresh piece of paper, and put yourself at the top of the tree. Now, have fun and fantasize about what you would like your legacy to be: What would the health picture of your children, your children's children, their children look like?

5. *What can you do now to make sure that future happens?* Steps you take today can influence your family's health for generations. If you've not yet had children, every bit of self-care that you show yourself now will pay dividends later in your children. If you already have kids, what changes can you model in your home so your kids will follow your lead? What changes can you make so you remind yourself to look around and enjoy the ride a little bit more?

As you read this chapter, think about your health goals and the goals you have for your family. Keep these sheets in a special folder, and refer to it often—it may just be OMD today, but these daily choices will have a ripple effect not only on your family, but on the entire world.

We Eat a *Lot* of Meat—and It's Killing Us

For all but the last seventy years, today's average American diet—high in saturated fat, sugar, and refined foods and low in fiber—would have been an unaffordable luxury for most humans. We now consume a whopping 180 pounds of meat per year per person. We eat like bloated, overindulgent kings and queens at every meal. And, fittingly, we're staggering under the burden of diseases like gout, heart disease, hypertension, type 2 diabetes, and obesity—often called "diseases of wealth."

For the first time in history, we are seeing a generation of children who will have a shorter life expectancy than their parents. Now it is the rule, rather than the exception, to develop one of these chronic diseases in your latter years. Dr. Barnard says many people assume that heart attacks or diabetes are caused by growing old, but they're really just caused by the accumulated damage of an unhealthy diet. "In the same way as lung cancer doesn't come because you're old, it comes because you accumulate so many cigarettes," says Dr. Barnard, "if we accumulate a whole lot of bacon strips, it adds up too."

What happens when a person develops diabetes or high blood pressure or high cholesterol and goes to visit their doctor? Most are immediately offered medication to "manage" their condition, to "control" the symptoms. How many doctors would ever hand you a prescription and say, "There you go—that pill will cure you."

They won't. Because they can't.

What if, instead of a prescription, your doctor handed you a cookbook?

Pills can't cure chronic disease—but diet can. Whole-food, plant-based diets have been linked[1] to:

- long-term, easier weight management[2]
- reduced blood sugar[3]
- reduced risk of cancer[4]
- reduced cholesterol[5]
- reduced blood pressure[6]
- reduced obesity[7]

- 🌐 reduced risk of dying from a heart attack[8]
- 🌐 reduced risk of overall mortality[9]
- 🌐 reduced need for medication[10]
- 🌐 reversal of advanced coronary artery disease[11,12]
- 🌐 reversal of type 2 diabetes[13]

An analysis published in the journal *Nature* found that switching to a whole-food, plant-based diet can reduce our risk of type 2 diabetes by over 40 percent; our risk of cancer by 13 percent; our risk of heart disease by over 20 percent; and our overall risk of illness by 18 percent.[14]

Eating a whole-food, plant-based diet automatically exposes us to a whole rainbow of foods. Jim likes to say, "When you go plant-based, you're cutting five species from your diet, but you're adding seventeen thousand." And it's true: you're basically trading a very small number of animal foods for a nearly endless variety of plant-based foods. That variety brings with it an impressive, ever-replenishing supply of disease-fighting phytochemicals and fiber that you simply cannot get from meat and dairy.

As you expand your food repertoire and eat more and different kinds of veggies (emphasis on "more," as you will be eating tons of food, rather happily), you start to realize just how amazing the vegetable and fruit world truly is. Mother Nature is a rock star. She knows how to make the healthiest foods irresistible. I mean, raspberries? Avocados? Fresh pineapple?

Mother Nature clearly knows what she's doing. Plant-based eating also increases our virility and fertility, improving our sex lives. That vixen! She's trying to romance us into eating the fruits of her labors so we can best reproduce and propagate the species. All we have to do is allow ourselves to be seduced by all those delicious, beautiful bountiful plants, and let nature take the wheel.

When we start to look at our most intractable health conditions, we see that animal products are at the center.

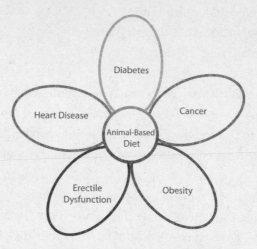

But when we switch to OMD and incorporate more plant-based foods, we find our health blossoms in a new way.

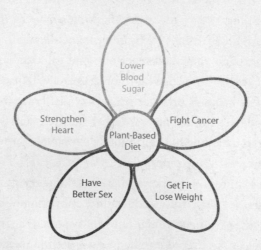

Let's dig down a little deeper into a few of the biggies here, to see how plant-based eating may not only help prevent, but could also reverse, some of the deadliest chronic diseases we face today.

A Plant-Based Diet Can . . .

- Give you shiny hair, glowing skin, and better breath
- Broaden your flavor palate
- Balance hormones and reduce PMS
- Decrease belly fat and stress hormone levels in the blood
- Greatly reduce risks of cancer, heart disease, and diabetes
- Help lower body weight
- Reduce risk of obesity among children
- Increase strength and performance in physical exercise
- Reduce inflammatory markers and symptoms of autoimmune disease, such as joint pain, stiffness, and muscle aches
- Reduce risk of cognitive decline
- Reduce risk of developing other degenerative diseases
- Improve your sexual vitality

OMD for Heart Health

My friend Brian Theiss is one of the last people you'd ever think would be at risk of heart disease. An Olympic weight lifter and strength and conditioning specialist at twenty-one, he had a terrible accident that left him paralyzed, disabled, and in chronic pain for a year. During that time, and due to the complexity of his physical and emotional state, coupled with the fact that there was no true physical therapy at the time for his condition, his neurosurgeon and he built his own physical therapy road back to recovery. On his way back to a normal life, he paid very close attention to his body and the instructions from his neurosurgeon. He also started interviewing doctors, scientists, and physiologists to get a better understanding of how to manage and deal with his new life. In his recovery, despite knowing that he will never recover fully, he went on to build a successful, comprehensive personal training business around the most efficient, effective way to recapture your health through the art and science of exercise.

Originally, I went to see Brian in 2008 because my knees were messed up. I wondered if I'd ever ski again. I'd been to a physical therapist and two doctors, and they'd all said it was likely I needed to have surgery. Well, enter Brian—he completely realigned my body, and now my knees are awesome. I'm still skiing extreme double-black-diamond slopes, and I'm pain-free.

Brian also taught me everything about fueling my workouts for recovery. Before I went plant-based, he had me on this program where I would eat crazy amounts of animal protein: yogurt with added whey for breakfast, handfuls of pumpkin seeds, and an 8-ounce chicken breast for dinner. After all my years of being concerned about *getting in that protein* while I was pregnant, that was no longer my problem— now I felt like I was seriously OD'ing on protein.

When Jim and I had our plant-based epiphany, I started eating plant-based yogurts and green smoothies with rice protein. Suddenly, I felt so much better—stronger, lighter, with crazy amounts of energy to spare. My body stopped fluctuating as much. Brian could plainly see that my muscle recovery was getting better, but he was skeptical.

Then one day while we were working out, he confessed that he'd had a scare with his blood pressure. The guy who'd taught me everything about working out efficiently, about how to eat to fuel, wasn't eating to live. Now it was my turn to help him.

I gave him *Forks Over Knives* and told him about how people who ate plant-based had significantly lower blood pressure than people who ate meat. About how carnitine—a component of red meat often found in bodybuilders' supplement regimens—can trigger inflammation in the arteries.

That was over six years ago; fast-forward to today, and his blood pressure is way down. He's feeling great. He looks a decade younger.

And now he's selling plant-based eating to all his clients. I want to say that I am so proud of Brian Theiss. Over thirty-one years of saving and changing the lives of more than nineteen thousand documented success cases, with his brilliant science mind, he took all my advice and did the research himself. Today he will tell you, that it was me, the student, who taught the master . . . and the master will forever be grateful.

Cardiovascular disease isn't just about the heart, of course—it starts in the arteries and blood vessels. And once again, cutting out beef is the way to make a major impact very quickly. When compared with people who eat red meat very often, people who eat less red meat and more vegetables have lower blood pressure, lower serum levels of LDL (the "bad" cholesterol), less thickening of the blood vessel walls, and less hardening of the arteries.[15] (And while red meat is the worst, bear in mind that chicken and salmon have the same amount of cholesterol as red meat. And shrimp has twice as much.)

Reduce Cholesterol and Inflammation

The walls of our blood vessels are protected by a lining of very sensitive cells called endothelial cells. When we eat too much animal fat, we can raise the level of LDL cholesterol in our blood. Those LDL molecules can burrow their way through tiny gaps between the endothelial cells and into the arterial walls. This disruption triggers our immune system to release inflammatory macrophage cells that come and suck up all that LDL, oxidizing it into stiff globs of plaque in the arterial walls. If we keep eating lots of saturated fats from animal products, those globs get bigger and bigger, eventually bulging out into the artery pathway and slowing blood flow. If they get angry and inflamed enough, they can even burst, triggering clots that can lead to heart attack and strokes.

Researchers have found a couple of markers that accurately reflect how disrupted these endothelial cells are—and both measures are directly tied to our diet. When you eat eggs, milk, liver, poultry, fish, or red meat—especially red meat—the carnitine and choline in those foods interact with a certain kind of bacteria in your gut to produce a chemical called TMAO (trimethylamine-N-oxide). The presence of TMAO in the blood has been strongly linked to heart attack, stroke, and chronic kidney disease. TMAO may even be the factor that triggers the activation of those macrophages that lead to arterial ruptures.

Just a single meal of animal products can spike inflammation and cause your arteries to stiffen. The link is so strong, in fact, that TMAO levels can be used as an accurate, independent predictor of our individual heart attack risk. People who are tested with high levels of TMAO have a four times greater risk of dying in the following five years.

On the flip side, the level of polyphenols (helpful plant chemicals such as antioxidants) in our system is another accurate predictor of our heart disease risk: the more vegetables we eat, the higher our level of polyphenols, and the lower the risk of heart disease. The guts of people who eat primarily whole-food, plant-based diets don't have the same bacteria that produce TMAO—so even if they happen to eat a piece of meat, their levels of the dangerous chemical would remain nearly negligible. The Nurses' Health Study, one of the largest and longest epidemiological studies in US history, found that those who ate the most fruits and vegetables had the lowest rates of cardiovascular disease; indeed, every extra serving of leafy greens they ate a day would decrease their risk by 11 percent.[16]

With OMD, you're increasing the amount of vegetables in your diet, but you don't have to give up your favorite foods. When you eat more plant-based whole foods, you're not only avoiding the processed foods, added sugars, oils, meats, and dairy that are linked to the oxidation of that LDL, you're replacing those foods with all kinds of glorious antioxidants and polyphenols that each have a unique role in repairing the endothelial cells, helping interrupt the macrophages from oxidizing all the LDL, and generally pumping the brakes on the entire inflammatory process. These healing bio-active chemicals protect the endothelium throughout your body, allowing the artery walls to heal and greatly reducing the likelihood of ruptures that can lead to stroke or heart attack. And with every plant-based OMD meal, you're also feeding beneficial bacteria in the gut that would further protect you from TMAO if you did eat a bit of meat.[17]

Reverse Heart Disease

In his landmark Lifestyle Heart Trial in 1990, Dr. Dean Ornish proved that a plant-based diet (combined with quitting smoking, moderate exercise, and reducing stress) could reverse heart disease. Over 80 percent of people who followed Dr. Ornish's program reversed their hardening of the arteries; even people with severe cases could experience a reversal within one year of starting his program. Those who followed the program lowered their LDL cholesterol by 40 percent after one year and by 20 percent after five years.[18,19] The control group who didn't follow the program was not as lucky—more than half of its members had *increased* levels of atherosclerosis after the study. The size of the lesions in the control group's cell walls increased, in the most severe cases by almost 7 percent, and shrank by 11 percent in the test group.

Now here we are, almost thirty years later, and these same results are still bearing out—and have only expanded. Consider the story of David Foster: At fifty-five, Foster had had a heart bypass, and now, two years later, at age fifty-seven, had 100 percent block-ages in his heart. His doctors told him his heart was so damaged, he needed a transplant—and worse, that even if he had the transplant, he could only expect to live another ten or eleven years.

Determined to save his own life, Foster signed up for Dr. Ornish's nine-week hospital-based outpatient Reversal Program in South Bend, Indiana; the program now features eight hours a week of instruction in whole-food, plant-based diet, as well as moderate exercise, stress management, and group support. After nine weeks, Foster was taken off the transplant list because his heart had improved so much. The Ornish Reversal Program is covered by Medicare and many insurances; 90 percent of patients who complete the program continue to follow it after one year. (Visit www.ornish.com/undo-it for more information.)

The power of plant-based nutrition is on my mind all the time. This past summer, I was standing behind this guy at a restaurant in Colorado, and I felt like I was watching someone order a whole spectrum of diseases. I pictured these subtitles over his head as he ordered: "I'd like some chicken wings [subtitle: *I'd like to order some heart disease for an appetizer*], and a filet mignon [*with an order of cancer as my main dish*], and a side of chili cheese fries [*with erectile dysfunction on the side*]."

Around the world, heart disease kills over seventeen million people a year—a number that the American Heart Association believes could grow to nearly twenty million in about ten years. Dr. Ornish proved, almost thirty years ago, that eating a plant-based diet can reverse heart disease in the span of a year. Since then, we've learned that our bodies show a measurable positive or negative response to *every single meal*, based on what's in it. We have the choice, every single time we sit down—do I want to hurt my heart with this meal, or heal it? With OMD, the choice couldn't be easier.

Prevent (and Reverse) Diabetes

I believe that most doctors are truly good individuals who want to help people, but most get woefully little nutrition training. In one survey of 106 medical schools, only 30 percent required aspiring doctors to take a separate nutrition course. On average, students received less than twenty-four total hours of nutritional instruction during their entire medical school career—and some received as little as *two hours*.[20]

We used to see our doctor every couple of weeks for some bug the kids picked up from school. Since we went plant-based, things that used to flatten the kids for a week or two now blow through in a couple of days. Jim and I haven't had a cold or flu in almost six years.

In 2012 I told the doctor we had gone plant-based. I talked about *Forks Over Knives* and *The China Study*, and told him I hoped he could support our decision. I was really surprised by how he responded. "All right, you can try that," he said, "but chances are you probably won't be able to maintain that kind of a lifestyle. It's going to be really hard." My jaw dropped. He shrugged. "That's why some doctors don't even recommend it—they don't think people are going to be able to stick with it."

Little did I know that that conversation did stick with someone, though. His nurse had been struggling with recurrent bouts of pancreatitis—every few months, she had to go into the hospital for about a week, couldn't eat anything, only IV and clear liquids. Horrifically painful. The next time I saw her to have my blood drawn, it was about a year later. She looked like a whole new person. I gushed, "Wow, you look completely different!"

She told me she'd lost twenty pounds and hadn't had a recurrence of pancreatitis at all. I was so surprised. She said, "Suzy, guess what? I went plant-based. I keep telling Dr. X, 'Look at me—I'm the poster child!' " Maybe her example will inspire him to have a little bit more faith in his patients! Give us a chance, doc. We might surprise you.

I was heartened by the nurse opting for a plant-based diet—as was her pancreas, clearly. If pancreatitis is not treated correctly, it can develop in many nasty directions—including diabetes. And we are certainly in the midst of an epidemic of diabetes in this country. According to the CDC, over one hundred million people in the United States have diabetes or prediabetes.[21] Nearly one in four adults who has diabetes doesn't even know. And while obesity is a risk factor for type 2 diabetes, eating meat, red meat in particular, appears to be a direct trigger for it. A study in *JAMA Internal Medicine* analyzed the meat intake of almost 150,000 men and women and found that those who'd started eating just a little bit more meat—an average of an extra half serving a day—had a 48 percent higher risk of having developed diabetes by the four-year check-in point. Those who ate heavily processed meats, such as hot dogs and bacon, had an even higher risk (51 percent). In contrast, those who'd trimmed a half serving from their daily intake had a 14 percent lower risk of developing diabetes.[22] Some epidemiological studies suggest that cultures in which children are given milk from A1 cows (the designation used for certain breeds, such as Holsteins, that are very common in the United States that were developed in Northern Europe) at an early age show a higher prevalence of type 1 diabetes.[23]

Plant-based diets protect against diabetes, and can even reverse it. The findings of the Adventist Health Studies, a set of epidemiological studies following 26,000 Seventh-day Adventists (who eat vegetarian or vegan as part of their religious observance) over twenty-one years, show that plant-based eaters have about half the risk of developing diabetes than the general population.[24] Another study found meat eaters' risk of developing diabetes over the course of seventeen years is closer to 74 percent higher than vegetarians' risk.[25]

These stats seem pretty dire, huh? But if I've learned anything from Dr. Barnard, it's the power of a plant-based diet to reverse diabetes. He conducted a randomized clinical trial in 2006, taking the standard American Diabetes Association guidelines and testing them against a low-fat, plant-based diet. In the resulting study, published in the ADA journal *Diabetes Care*, he showed that following a low-fat, plant-based diet for twenty-two weeks helped people reduce their HbA1c (a measure of long-term blood sugar control) by 1.23 points versus 0.38 points in the ADA group. The plant-based group also dropped twice as much weight—14.3 pounds versus 6.8 pounds—and over 40 percent were able to reduce their medications (versus 26 percent in the ADA group).[26] Overall, a clearly superior outcome.

Since then, many important studies have shown similar results. In 2017, a study published in the *Journal of the American College of Nutrition* found that people with type 2 diabetes were almost twice as successful at losing weight on a vegetarian diet compared to those on the standard European diabetes diet—and, after six months, the vegetarians showed much less fat inside their muscles, a sign that they'd made a lasting change in their glucose and fat metabolism and had developed leaner muscle.[27]

Dr. Barnard told us the story of a patient from Canada who weighed 320 pounds. The man's doctor had said to him, "I can tell you exactly where this is going to go. You're going to end up with diabetes and you'll end up with all these problems." The man had heard about the work Dr. Barnard was doing, so he went and asked for Dr. Barnard's help. Well, the man got animal products off his plate and loaded up with healthful foods, and about a year later, he'd lost 160 pounds. "His diabetes was gone," recalls Dr. Barnard. "He was really reclaiming health."

Let's hear it for plant power!

Have Better Sex

There's something that Jim always makes sure that I remember to tell people: plant-based eaters have great sex.

OK, I'm blushing—Jim is my husband, and we are plant-based, after all. So, let me put that more politely: men who follow plant-based eating patterns tend to have substantially lower rates of heart disease, and erectile dysfunction is one of the classic early warning signs of clogged arteries.

Men who have heart disease and diabetes—two conditions closely associated with heavy meat and dairy consumption—have much higher rates of erectile dysfunction. I'm talking 35 percent of men with high blood pressure, 42 percent of men with high cholesterol, and up to *85 percent of men with diabetes* have some degree of erectile dysfunction.[28] (And bear in mind: These are only the men who have reported erectile dysfunction—many others live with it and are too embarrassed to mention it.)

A guy in his forties who's having trouble getting an erection has a fiftyfold increased chance of a cardiac event—that's a *5,000 percent* greater risk. And a whopping 40 percent of men over age forty suffer from erectile dysfunction. And they're not alone—studies have found that women with arterial plaque also have significantly decreased arousal and ability to orgasm.

Here's something that a lot of guys just haven't caught onto yet: plant-based eating is the new Viagra! That's right, my friends: Hot sex, cool planet! Sadly, guys have been missing out. Statistics show that men eat 57 percent more meat than women, twice the protein they need.[29] That's not a big shock considering that one study found that men are perceived to be 35 percent more masculine when they eat meat.[30]

But the truth is, going green is *studly*! A 2017 review published in the journal *Biomedicine & Pharmacotherapy* looked at all the studies on erectile dysfunction and plant-based diets in the past forty-four years, and found *ten separate chemical pathways* through which the antioxidant polyphenols in plants help to reverse erectile dysfunction.[31]

I'm hoping that we can wean men off meat and get them to see the light—because what could be sexier than a guy who's stronger, leaner, and has more endurance? Someone who has a . . . heart that can easily pump all night.

Science tells us that the more men eat meat, the more quickly they lose their erectile function. In the documentary *The Game Changers*, for which Jim and I are among the executive producers, the crew shot an experiment conducted by Dr. Aaron Spitz, lead delegate of urology for the American Medical Association. He took three college athletes and fed them burritos over two consecutive nights. The first night, one player had a burrito with organic free-range chicken; one had organic grass-fed beef; and one had organic pork. The second night, all three of them ate a plant-based burrito made with alternative chicken, beef, and pork. (The chef was gratified when one guy said, "If you'd told me I had meat tonight and plant-based meat yesterday, I couldn't tell the difference.")

On each night, the men were fitted with a device called a Rigiscan, which measured the circumference of their penis while they slept. The night the men ate the bean burritos instead of the meat burritos, Dr. Spitz told them their penises were an average of 10.4 percent (ahem) harder and bigger, and they experienced a 364 percent increase in the number of nighttime erections. After the meat-based meals, they'd had an average of 11 minutes of erections overnight; after the plant-based meals, they'd had 45 minutes of erections. As James Wilks, plant-based Ultimate Fighter and narrator of *The Game Changers*, says, "A single meal can make a *major* difference, even in a young, healthy body."

If men start to have erectile dysfunction, it means their arteries are clogged and they have heart disease. ED is the canary in the coal mine. In *Eating You Alive*, a documentary in which Jim and I recently appeared, Dr. Evan Allen, a urologist in Henderson, Nevada, made the stakes brutally clear: "ED to a urologist is erectile dysfunction; to a cardiologist, it means something else: early death."

Lose Weight

Honestly, about nine out of ten of the "before and after" stories I hear from people after they go plant-based involve seemingly magically or effortlessly getting to or staying at a healthy weight. Either they lose weight or maintain a healthy weight more easily, and perhaps best of all, they're able to completely stop worrying about it. One review in *Nutrition Reviews* of eighty-seven studies found that plant-based diets require zero exercise to achieve a weight loss of about one pound per week—a very healthy, sustainable, maintainable rate any doctor could love. (Not that you shouldn't exercise, of course!) The study suggested that part of the effectiveness comes from the way our bodies react to plant-based meals in contrast to animal products. After eating animal products, our bodies tend to store the calories as fat. In contrast, after eating plant-based meals, the body tends to start burning calories immediately, right after we eat.[32]

If weight loss was your only metric, of all the possible "weight-loss" diets out there, plant-based eating appears to top every single one. In a cross-sectional study of over seventy thousand people published in the *Journal of the Academy of Nutrition and Dietetics*, researchers examined the eating patterns of five groups: meat eaters, semi-vegetarians (occasional meat eaters), pesco vegetarians (vegetarians who eat fish), lacto-ovo vegetarians (vegetarians who consume dairy), and vegans. Surprise: Vegans had the lowest average BMI, while meat eaters had the highest. Meat eaters ate way less plant proteins, fiber, beta-carotene, and magnesium—but much more fat of all kinds (saturated, trans, omega-6, and omega-3). They also had a whopping 33 percent obesity rate, while vegans had a rate of only 9.4 percent. Researchers noted that the obesity rate seemed directly proportional to the amount of animal products in a person's diet: occasional meat eaters had a 24 percent rate of obesity, pesco vegetarians had 17.9 percent, and lacto-ovo vegetarians had 16.7 percent. All the groups ate roughly the same number of calories, about 2,000 per day—the biggest difference was the *source* of those calories.[33]

When a European study followed people with essentially the same types of eating patterns for five years, researchers found those who switched to a plant-based eating approach during that time gained the least amount of weight.[34] Epidemiologists have found the same patterns applied to children: vegetarian kids are consistently leaner, and the differences in the BMI between meat eaters and plant-based kids became more pronounced during adolescence. (A perfect time to help kids fend off that childhood obesity we're all so nervous about.[35])

Perhaps the best part about losing weight by going plant-based is the total, utter simplicity of the "rules." There's no calorie counting. Needn't be any fussy nutrient ratios. True, if you have a specific health concern (such as heart disease, diabetes, or cancer), you might want to follow a more structured plant-based program to ensure you get the best information and you can follow specifically designed nutrient ratios (and I'll suggest many such books in the OMD Resource Well, page 314). Overall, though, calorie for calorie, just opting for whole-food, plant-based eating will automatically give you more fiber, antioxidants, vitamins, and minerals, and a whole lot less fat, packing some serious nutrition into each bite.[36] If you're just looking to drop a few pounds and get off the weight roller coaster for good, there are basically only two rules: 1) eat food that grows from the ground; and 2) try not to eat food that comes from a box, bottle, or can. Trust your appetite, follow (and honor) your cravings, enjoy your meals, and eat until you're satisfied and energized, and believe me—those miraculous plants will do much of the weight loss work for you.

My former manager, Davien, is the epitome of trusting the process and keeping things simple. "I'm not a very complicated vegan.

I'm not the kind of person whose commitment is based on saving the world or saving animals," she says. "It's all about feeling better."

Get Buff

Some of my family are truck-driving, jerky-eating carnivores. Inevitably, in the early days of our plant-based conversion, we'd be at some family gathering, about to eat, and I'd get the evergreen question asked of every plant-based eater: "How do you get your protein?"

I'll discuss protein more in chapter 4, "Prepare to OMD," but for now, let's tackle the muscle-bound version of this question. Men, in particular, seem very concerned that they will not be able to get enough protein to support their muscle mass.

Nothing could be further from the truth.

I will never forget the day my entire family got collectively (and humorously) schooled on the protein question. Just a couple of months after Jim and I went plant-based, we were at our farm in Oklahoma for our annual Amis family reunion, out on my sister Page's party barge boat. Page had not yet gone plant-based, so she made one of her famous "lake sandwiches": a long, fat loaf of French bread smeared with mayo and layered with lettuce, tomato, three kinds of cheese, salami, ham, and turkey. I had never been a huge fan of the sandwich, but now it was a hard no-go for my whole family.

Well, cue the teasing.

My son Quinn, nine at the time, had taken all the meat and cheese out and was about to throw it overboard. My eldest brother, Dave, grabbed it and came right over to me, dangled the meat really close to my face, and said, "This is so good. Don't you want a bite?" Then he tipped his head back and ate it in one bite. So gross. Typical big brother.

Then Dave turned to Quinn and said, "How are you going to get your protein, young man?"

I am eternally grateful that Ben, our nanny, was there with us that day. Ben had gone plant-based with us and is just about the buffest specimen you will ever see. When he heard that comment, he jumped up, went right over to Dave, pointed at his twelve-pack, and asked, "Do I look like I need more protein?"

Class dismissed.

I truly believe we are on the cusp of plant-based athletes being the norm, not the exception. If you want to see dozens of elite level competitors who've only improved their performance since making the switch, check out the documentary *The Game Changers*—these world-class professional athletes are sterling examples of how plant-based nutrition can fuel extraordinary levels of physical performance. (For visual proof, check out the photos of family and friends—including Ben's crazy abs—at https://omdfortheplanet.com/media-center/gallery.) A study published in the *American Journal of Clinical Nutrition* looked at the health records and diet diaries of nearly three thousand people, from teens all the way to the elderly, to determine which type of protein—plant or animal—was better at building and preserving muscle mass. The verdict? A perfect tie. Zero difference.

So if your sole focus and concern is building muscle, eating plant-based is a one-to-one swap with eating meat. But when you factor in all the hormones, antibiotics, heavy metals, endotoxins, and other garbage in animal products (all of which increase your inflammation and decrease performance), and the fact that plant proteins help you keep your weight on an even keel much easier—plus, oh yeah, the fate of the planet—that balance starts to tip just a little.

Perhaps Dr. Barnard says it best: "So many people have the idea that protein has to come from meat. Well, if the meat came from the cow, what was the cow eating? That cow is a vegan.

"If you take the biggest bull, the fastest stallion with those rippling muscles, the biggest elephant, the tallest giraffe, they're getting their protein entirely from plant sources. And so if you add up the protein in beans and grains and vegetables, it's more than enough for you, including top-level athletes. You're going to get the protein you need."

Or, Jim adds, "Consider the gorilla—it has the closest intestinal tract to humans, and they are fully plant-based. A gorilla could rip your arm out of the socket and beat you to death with the bloody stump." Personally, I have found that plant-based folks are a little more peaceful than that, but it's instructive to consider.

Cure Cancer

Before she went plant-based herself, my sister Page always wanted my kids to have those sandwiches at the lake. There were years when I just looked the other way; I didn't want to become dogmatic about it. Besides, I knew there were sentimental things the kids missed—like lemon chess pie or creamed corn (before Mom made her "vay-gan" version)—and I understood the struggle. I hated that my siblings would tease me. I didn't want my kids to feel like the odd ones out.

That's the most challenging thing for me when I go home to Oklahoma—watching people I love eat meat and dairy and knowing it's not good for them. It's tough. I rarely say anything, but it's tough. I remember going home during the last two years of my dad's life, and seeing my mom's fridge full of cheese and yogurt. But then she also had a raw vegan cookbook on her shelf. Sometimes she's open to talking about it; sometimes she's not. We all get there in our own time. I have to realize there's nothing I can say, and they have to figure it out on their own. To date she has broken both hips and her pelvis. I wonder if this would have happened if she were plant-based.

Since that first summer, Page has gone plant-based too—but an even bigger wake-up call came when her husband, Ken, was diagnosed with kidney cancer early last year.

The winter after our transition to plant-based eating, I'd sent everyone on our Christmas gift list what affectionately became known as "the bag"—a canvas shoulder bag filled with books and DVDs about plant-based eating. The first year, we focused on books with the health angle. The second year, the environmental angle. And while I know that Jim and I had only the best intentions, I fully own the fact that—let's just say—it was not "well received" by everyone in our family and friend circle. Page's husband, Ken, for example, was not having it. Not any of it. And then he had his cancer scare—and he went fully plant-based.

MY OMD STORY

Ken Beatty

When Jim and Suzy started sending out that gift package—well, I just rejected it. I'd never even heard the word *vegan*. I thought, *There's no way we can do that in Oklahoma*.

Then, on October 16, 2016, my mom passed away. She had cirrhosis of the liver, but she didn't drink. I thought, *I don't want to die like that*.

I went in to see my doctor to get some blood tests. He reassured me that cirrhosis of the liver isn't hereditary in any way, took my blood, and sent me on my way.

A few weeks later, he called and said, "Hey, why don't you come in for an ultrasound?" *No problem*, I thought. *I'm invincible*. I did a few more tests, and in January, I got the call: "Ken, you got cancer."

They took my kidney out on January 24, 2017. I never had any symptoms. It was just extreme luck that I happened to go get that test when I did. I'd had my elbow and knee operated on, I'd had two spinal discs replaced. None of that really bothered me. But when they started pulling organs out—that bothered me.

When I first heard the word *cancer*, I was invincible. Then I was looking for what caused my cancer, and the truth is, it could have been a million things. Now I know that the majority of kidney disease comes from your diet: milk, cheese, eggs, processed foods. Inflammation, fungus, infections—we all have this stuff inside of us. Most of us just don't know it.

That's when I was finally ready to eat plant-based. I just had no cravings for junk anymore. I started avoiding sugar, eating smaller portions. And always plant-based.

I'm a 35-inch waist now. (Before, I was a 38 or 40.) I'm a big guy—I started at 258, and after about six months, I'm down to 199. Now if I eat something non-plant-based, I'm pretty hard on myself. Because now I know I'm not invincible—you never know what is going to be the thing that triggers this again.

These days, Ken is a new man. Now, bear in mind, Ken went way beyond OMD—he went fully plant-based, which helped him do a complete one-eighty in just six months. He's constantly reading and looking online for cool new information. Now we talk about the gut microbiome, herbal preparations, apple cider vinegar. After knowing him for all these years, watching his transformation is nothing short of extraordinary. (Now he proudly says, "I used to be fatty Daddy and now I'm skinny Kenny!") I'm so glad he caught his cancer so soon. And I'm so glad we're all on this journey together. Plant-based eating is changing my family's life—and not a moment too soon. (You can see before and after photos of Ken and many other plant-based transformations at https://omdfortheplanet.com /get-started/success-stories.)

Cancer is the number two killer (second only to heart disease) of Americans of all ages and demographics. The disease in all its myriad forms has become so ingrained in our universal experience that the phrase "the cure for cancer" has become shorthand for "the highest possible good one can do." But, increasingly, researchers are discovering that curing—or at least reducing the instance of cancer—could be as simple as changing our diets.

Meat, particularly red meat, has been linked to many cancers, most strongly rectal, breast, prostate, stomach, and colon cancers, via a variety of pathways. When meat is processed or cooked, it produces carcinogenic compounds (heterocyclic amines, or HCAs, and polycyclic aromatic hydrocarbons, or PAH, among others) that increase cancer risk. HCAs are produced during the cooking of beef, pork, poultry, and even that favorite so-called "healthy" meat, fish. Equally alarming are the nitrates and nitrites used in processed meat. The World Health Organization (WHO) has determined that for each 50 gram portion of processed meat (the equivalent of one hot dog or four strips of bacon) that we eat daily, our risk of colorectal cancer goes up by 18 percent. WHO now classifies processed meat as Group 1 carcinogen, the same class as cigarettes, asbestos, and plutonium. Sadly, digestive cancers, once thought to be a disease of the elderly, are dramatically on the rise among twenty- to forty-nine-year-olds.

Another troubling substance is insulin-like growth factor (IGF), a hormone in milk that's intended to help young calves grow, but that can be extra dangerous for adult humans. When we drink milk, it stimulates our body's endogenous production of IGF-1, which can lead to extra cell proliferation.[37] Yet another concern: Heme iron (found in animal foods) is absorbed faster than nonheme iron (found in plant foods), and excess amounts can increase levels of inflammation and heighten colon cancer risk,[38] in addition to reducing cells' sensitivity to insulin, raising the risk of diabetes.

And keep in mind that about 70 percent of all medically important antibiotics sold in the United States are used in raising meat and dairy,[39] given to livestock to promote growth and prevent widespread illnesses in their packed industrial farms, which sets the stage for widespread antibiotic resistance that could potentially kill many people. When any one hamburger can be made with meat from as many as one hundred different cows, any resistant infections would become very hard to trace—and contain. We are only just learning the extent to which this abuse of these powerful, life-saving drugs might have already altered our collective microbiome, leaving our guts extremely vulnerable to virulent bacteria that can weaken our immune systems, ramp up inflammation,[40] and potentially leave us unable to summon our healing power when powerful diseases like cancer strike.[41]

What Is the Microbiome?

You may have heard people tossing around the word *microbiome* recently. You may have a vague sense of it as the balance of good and bad bacteria in your gut—but it's so much more. The microbiome is the sum total of all the genes of the microbes that live in and on our bodies, which help us digest our food, boost our immune system, fight off pathogens, and more. For every single gene we have, our microbe population has one hundred. While our human genetic material—our genome—is fixed from birth, our microbiome adapts constantly in reaction to the environment. Most of these changes are beneficial and keep us healthy and operating well, but when we overuse antibiotics, we can damage our microbes' ability to adapt and protect us— and those formerly protective microbes can become sitting ducks for pathogens and disease. By eating lots of plant-based fiber (*prebiotics*) along with fermented foods filled with beneficial anti-inflammatory bacteria (*probiotics*), we help strengthen our healthy microbiome population so it can gang up and crowd out the bad guys.

In contrast, plant-based eating does basically the opposite, in basically every way. Plant foods displace the environmental toxins that concentrate in animal tissue, build up our immune system's resilience, and feed our healthy gut bacteria with phytochemicals that actually *reduce* the risk of cancer. Studies show that plant-based eaters are 20 percent less likely to die from any cancer, and 50 to 60 percent less likely to die from pancreatic, lymphatic, or blood cancers.[42] Plant-based women are 34 percent less likely to develop reproductive cancers (breast, cervical, ovarian) than female meat eaters.[43] All those glorious, immune-boosting antioxidants in plants have been proven to fight cancer in so many ways—they stop tumors from growing, help the body detoxify from carcinogens, prevent errant cell growth, and even block cancer formation before it can start.[44]

And don't forget: Plants are our only source of fiber, which feeds the beneficial bacteria that produce anticancer short-chain fatty acids in our digestive system. When our digestive systems are "regular," that means fiber is doing its job, helping collect all those toxins, fats, cholesterol, and hormones in the digestive tract and whisking them out of the body. Adios, cancer.

OMD AND PUBLIC HEALTH

Going plant-based doesn't just help the health of your family—these effects will ripple out into the health of the wider world. With OMD and a plant-based diet forecasted over the long term, on a global scale, we will start to see:

- **Less antibiotic resistance:** By reducing the use of antibiotics in the food supply, we can protect the effectiveness of these life-saving medicines.

- **Protection of indigenous cultures:** From the Ulithi in the South Pacific to the Kayapo in the Brazilian rain forest, these peoples' health, safety, and entire way of life have been endangered by the effects of animal agriculture on the climate—and reversing that trend could help stall these changes and help them rebuild.

🌍 **Reduction of chronic disease epidemics**: The steady rise of lifestyle diseases linked to animal product consumption, such as heart disease, diabetes, and cancer, can be reduced dramatically with plant-based diets.

🌍 **Reversal of downward longevity trajectory**: By improving our chronic disease outlook, we could help reverse the trend of a shortened average life span.

🌍 **Generation-level epigenetic changes**: These positive health changes will limit vulnerability to genetic risks of disease and continue to compound with each successive generation of plant-based eaters.[45]

🌍 **Universal food security**: By using proteins derived from plants rather than animals, we can feed ten times as many people with the same resources.

OMD Grows Stronger Bodies and Minds

In 2012, when I first saw *Forks Over Knives* and realized how we've all been misled for so many years, I was distraught. Until that moment, I truly believed we were feeding our own kids (and all the children at MUSE) the best way possible—grass-fed beef, free-range chicken, organic cheese and yogurt, the highest-quality organic milk, all that stuff. In one day, I went from, "Man, we are doing a great job" to "Oh my goodness, I'm killing my family! I'm killing myself! I'm killing all these kids at school! And I am killing the planet!"

I felt so lied to. I didn't know whom to trust. It was time to take action.

When Rebecca and I decided to enlist the help of what we would later term "the OMD brain trust," we were so fortunate to have the help of Dr. Neal Barnard and Dr. Dean Ornish. Parents were so confused and concerned about the plant-based lunch plan that Dr. Barnard prepared the following information sheet about plant-based nutrition for us to share with the entire school community. Dr. Barnard's steady confidence and unassailable credibility were crucial in helping us win over the parent community. I'm so grateful for all he's done to help MUSE and OMD. He's a genius.

NUTRITION POWER FOR CHILDREN BUILDING STRONG BODIES AND MINDS

by Dr. Neal Barnard, Physicians Committee for Responsible Medicine*

Nutrition is essential for physical and cognitive health. Unfortunately, modern life leads many people to neglect good nutrition. Young people especially are not getting the nutrients they need.

The Centers for Disease Control and Prevention described the problem this way:

"Most U.S. residents, including children, consume too few fruits and vegetables. In 2007 to 2010, 60 percent of children aged one to eighteen did not meet U.S. Department of Agriculture Food Patterns fruit intake recommendations, and 93 percent did not meet vegetable recommendations. Because of the benefits of eating fruits and vegetables and because childhood dietary patterns are associated with food patterns later in life, encouraging children to eat more fruits and vegetables is a public health priority."[46]

* Dr. Neal Barnard, MD, FACC, is an adjunct associate professor of medicine at the George Washington University School of Medicine and Health Sciences in Washington, DC, president of the Physicians Committee for Responsible Medicine, and founder of Barnard Medical Center. Dr. Barnard prepared a version of this information sheet for parents of MUSE students who were transitioning to plant-based lunches with the OMD program in 2012–2013.

Studies show that children whose diets emphasize plant-based foods grow as tall or taller than their meat-eating friends, and gain a measure of protection from the health risks that await many young people as they reach adulthood: obesity, diabetes, hypertension, and heart disease, among others.[47,48]

Decades ago, researchers discovered that children following plant-based diets had much higher average IQs, compared with children following omnivorous diets. In a Tufts University study, children on plant-based diets had an average 16-point advantage over other children on standardized IQ testing.[49] Conversely, British researchers found that children with higher IQs are more likely to select plant-based diets in adulthood.[50]

Investing in nutrition early in life can also help protect brain function later on. In middle age and later life, many people have problems with memory, reasoning, and reaction time. In a Loma Linda University study, cognitive loss was not nearly as severe among people following plant-based diets, compared with people following meat-based diets.[51] Plant-derived foods skip most of the saturated fat that has been shown to be related to brain problems in older age.[52] And many plant-based foods are rich in natural vitamin E, which has shown protective effects for brain function.[53,54]

A few nutrients merit special mention:

Glucose. The brain runs on glucose. Fruit, grains, beans, and starchy vegetables are healthful sources, releasing glucose gradually into the bloodstream. These sources have tremendous advantages over processed foods, as they also provide valuable vitamins, minerals, fiber, antioxidants, and phytochemicals.

Essential amino acids. The brain also needs small amounts of amino acids—the building blocks of protein—to produce neurotransmitters. All the essential amino acids are found in plant foods, without the saturated fat and cholesterol that are common to animal-derived products.

Essential fatty acids. Two fats are essential for the body and brain in trace amounts: alpha-linolenic acid (ALA) and linoleic acid (LA). ALA is an omega-3 fatty acid that is abundant in plant-based foods, such as walnuts, oats, beans, and flaxseed. Leafy greens are a particularly interesting source. While they do not contain much fat overall, the fat they do have is proportionately high in ALA. Broccoli, for example, gets not quite 10 percent of its calories from fat, but a large proportion of that fat is ALA. Broccoli is also about one-third protein.

In the human body, enzymes lengthen ALA to produce other omega-3s, called EPA and DHA, which play roles in brain function. These enzymes are slowed down when people consume large quantities of other fats. So it makes sense to take advantage of healthful ALA-containing foods, while avoiding overdoing it with fatty foods in general.

Some people get omega-3 fats from fish. However, fish also contain cholesterol, saturated fat, and, in some cases, worrisome amounts of mercury and other environmental toxins that pose dangers to growing children.

Some people also take EPA and DHA supplements in hopes of improving brain function, although their benefits are not yet established. These supplements are available in both vegan and nonvegan brands.

Eating for Energy

Blood circulation is essential for delivering oxygen and nutrients to all parts of the body. However, animal fats tend to make the blood more viscous ("thicker"), which increases blood pressure and reduces blood flow. A low-fat, plant-based diet has the opposite effect, reducing blood viscosity and improving blood flow, which not only promotes heart health, but also energy levels.[55] Many athletes, especially endurance athletes, are now using plant-based diets for a competitive edge.

The Advantage for Your Child

Many children get too much sugar, too much fat, and too much salt in their processed-food, animal-centered diets. Having one well-planned plant-based meal each day means that they will boost their intakes of the foods that are so often lacking: fresh vegetables, fruits, legumes, and whole grains. Good nutrition does more than help children grow. It gives them lifelong health advantages.

MY OMD STORY

Allison Braine

When I came to teach kindergarten at MUSE, I had already been a vegetarian for about five years. Then I started eating the fully plant-based OMD, and I really embraced it. Before, when I was vegetarian it was for health reasons. I wanted to take good care of myself, but now my mind was open to thinking about the animals. Going fully plant-based just meant giving up those few things—so it was a no-brainer. I like testing my body and feeling healthy, so I dropped eggs and cheese. I thought I might feel tired eating fully plant-based, but I didn't.

I've seen parents react to the idea of a plant-based diet. They're pretty vocal about it—there is both concern and excitement. The OMD program can be helpful for families that are curious and want to try eating plant-based at home. A lot of the parents embraced the one meal a day concept because they like that they don't feel pressure to be vegan. They're also happy that the kids are exposed to that one plant-based meal. A lot of the families are not vegan, but everyone practices one meal a day.

We have a lot of opportunities to talk to the kids about plant-based eating, whether through garden education, composting, or just eating the different foods. It's so nice to hear four- to five-year-olds talking about and developing their understanding of food at this age. One kid will say that they eat chicken at home, and another kid will explain that he doesn't eat meat because, "I don't want my teeth to hurt animals!" So cute. If someone brings in a treat for birthdays, or if we have a bake sale, you have these little kids asking if something is vegan. Some students who are plant-based really enjoy the meat substitutes. Other plant-based students don't even like the fake meat, they just prefer straight raw vegetables. Because the kids are all exposed to this one meal a day, and all of the surrounding discussions, they'll be more open and able to make conscious choices as they grow up.

One of the parents shared the most hilarious story. They were in the grocery story when her little son started throwing a tantrum because she had promised him *tofu*! Most kids are like, "I want a cookie!" or "give me this chocolate!" She was a little embarrassed, but couldn't help cracking up because her kid was there screaming, "You promised you'd buy us tofu!"

Tackling the Four Ns

Researchers from Lancaster University in the UK analyzed the reasons why people eat meat and found that 90 percent of them professed to the "four Ns" of meat-eating: they consider eating meat to be "necessary, natural, normal, and nice."[56] Social psychologist Melanie Joy coined the term *carnism* to describe the eating of meat as the corollary to the word *vegan*—both are simple descriptors of the basis of each person's diet, but it highlights how vegans are considered the oddity. "People are socialized not only to believe that eating animals is normal, natural, and necessary, but that not eating animals is abnormal, unnatural, and unnecessary," she says. Let's look at the four Ns one by one.

Is meat necessary? Processed meat has been designated a carcinogen by WHO, and diets that are rich in meat are associated with increased rates of heart disease and other major chronic diseases. We *can* digest meat—but we are also able to digest paper, mud, and other nonnutritive-yet-still-edible substances. Bottom line: We can get all the nutrients we need from plants—and we can supplement for the very few nutrients that come in short supply (see "Getting All the Nutrition Bases Covered" on page 110 for more info).

"There's no convincing literature saying that modern societies get better when people eat more meat," says Dr. David Katz, founding director of the Yale-Griffin Prevention Research Center. But "there's overwhelming evidence to say that the prevailing ailments in modern societies get better when people eat more vegetables, fruits, whole grains, beans, lentils, nuts, and seeds." Large populations of plant-based eaters are among the healthiest on the planet.

Is meat natural? "You can't say that humans are adapted to eat grain-fed beef, let alone pepperoni," says Katz. "There was no Paleolithic pastrami, for crying out loud." If someone is invoking a native diet as a reason to eat meat, Dr. Katz would like to issue a challenge: "Get a bow and arrow or a spear, and get out there, go the miles, wait in the woods, and have venison for dinner tonight."

Is meat normal? We've been raised to think that meat is "the point" of the meal—the sun around which all the (usually vegetable-based) side dishes orbit. But, if we step back and think of it, we can recognize that this is just our mental habit. We can consciously redefine what "normal" is at any time. Melanie Joy says that meat is just accepted as a given, so the idea of eating meat has become invisible, and the choice *not* to eat meat is seen as the exception: "There's vegans and vegetarians, and then there's everyone else." But for most of the world, for most of human history, eating meat at this level was not normal. At most, it was eaten sparingly, as Dr. Mark Hyman refers to it, as "condimeat"—akin to a seasoning on top of a plant-based meal rather than the foundation of the meal itself. Unfortunately, our "normal" consumption of meat is becoming the norm around the world—and the trajectory is truly unsustainable.

Is meat nice? We might like the sensation of biting down into a burger—that might feel satisfying and familiar, and "nice." But with all the new advancements in meat analogues—such as Alpha Foods, Hungry Planet Beef, and burgers from Impossible Foods and Beyond Meat—we're getting closer and closer to that mouthfeel with every iteration. Perhaps, when weighing it against all the other mitigating factors, it's time to say that feeling is not quite equivalent to the destruction it represents. We are compassionate people who have been taught to dissociate from the cow that burger came from. We don't like to think about the way animals are raised because, no, it really isn't nice. "The way we generate meat today is cruel and unbelievably costly to the environment," says Dr. Katz. "And because it adulterates the meat and changes the nutritional composition, it makes meat bad for health too."

Instead of thinking about OMD as "giving up" animal products for one meal a day, think about everything you *get* as you eat a more plant-based diet—a wider variety of colors, flavors, and textures, and an endless world of experimentation and food combinations; guilt-free and automatic weight loss and/or management; all that smooth skin and shiny hair and those sparkling eyes; an endless supply of vitamins, minerals, and soluble and insoluble fiber; and all those glorious antioxidants that can tamp down runaway inflammation and keep your innards humming along happily. (Did I mention hot sex, cool planet?)

Live a Longer Life

What's the ultimate benefit of a life lived eating a plant-based diet?

A longer and healthier life.

Isn't that what we're all hoping for? A few more years with the grandkids. A few more adventures with our honey. A few more books read (or written!), movies watched (or made!). More of the essence of why we are all here.

And to know we could *all* get that by making small choices that also help the planet in a major way? No matter what balance sheet you're looking at, OMD is a pretty good deal.

In a Harvard University study of 130,000 patients over thirty years, researchers found that swapping just 3 percent of your animal protein for plant protein—3 percent!—dramatically reduces your risk of death. The researchers found:

- If you swap 3 percent of your unprocessed red meat for plant protein, you're 12 percent less likely to die.
- If you swap 3 percent of your egg protein for plant protein, you're 19 percent less likely to die.
- If you swap 3 percent of your processed red meat for plant protein, you're 34 percent less likely to die.

They found that eating more plant-based foods could protect you from dying early even if (especially if) you smoke, drink every day, are overweight or obese, and/or are sedentary.[57] Although I'm certainly not telling you to start smoking or sitting around all day! But if you're going to give up one life-shortening habit, your odds seem to get a bit better when you make it meat.

We lengthen and shorten our lives in a million ways, large and small, throughout every day. We might cuss and fume at rush-hour traffic, or we use the time to listen to a book on tape. We might choose to stand far away from, or right next to, the exhaust of a city bus. We might opt to watch television from the treadmill or the elliptical instead of the couch.

Every meal is also a chance to choose. Will you choose more inflammation, or less? More endotoxins, or less?

More cancer-fighting, heart-and-brain-protecting, microbiome-feeding fiber and polyphenols, or less?

In essence, every single meal is a new chance to choose a shorter life, or a longer one. Repeated day after day, these small choices become your destiny.

Thirty years ago, we learned from Dr. Dean Ornish that what we ate could reverse heart disease. Now, thirty years later, Dr. Ornish and his esteemed colleagues, including Nobel laureate Dr. Elizabeth Blackburn, are on the cusp of proving that what we eat can extend our lives, starting on a genetic level.

You may have heard of telomeres, the protective caps on the ends of our chromosomes that guard against damage. When we're young, these telomeres are long, but they gradually get worn down over the course of our lives. Shorter telomeres are associated with chronic diseases such as heart disease, dementia, and cancer—and shorter lives.

We used to think a telomere was like a wick of a candle—burn them down, and they're gone. But it turns out there's an enzyme called telomerase that helps extend and regrow telomeres. Now the only question for Dr. Ornish and his team was, how do you increase telomerase?

With funding from the Department of Defense and the National Institutes of Health, Dr. Ornish conducted a small, five-year pilot study to answer that question.[58] Can we increase the amount of telomerase in our cells, and thereby lengthen the life span of our chromosomes, just from the choices we make?

For five years, a group of ten men in their sixties followed Dr. Ornish's program: thirty minutes of exercise a day, one hour of yoga and meditation a day, one session of group therapy once a week, and—of course—a whole-food, plant-based diet.

A control group of twenty-five just went along with their normal lives.

After five years, those guys who'd just gone along with their normal regimes showed a predictable sign of "aging"—their telomeres were now 3 percent shorter than they'd been at the start of the study.

But the test group?

In the men who followed the program, their telomeres were *10 percent longer* than they'd been five years before. That's right—they appeared to not only have stopped their body's aging, they'd turned the clock back. The "aging" process that had previously been presumed to be unavoidable, a one-way street to a literal dead end, was now looking like a largely optional, totally reversible process—much like heart disease had seemed thirty years before.

The best finding of the study? We don't have to wait five years to see those kinds of results. After only three months on the program, the men's bodies were starting to produce significantly more telomerase. Dr. Ornish and his colleagues were able to watch this reverse-aging in real time.

In a way, we have already known the punch line to this study. Plant-based people live longer, full stop. An analysis of six large studies on hundreds of thousands of people, published in the *American Journal of Clinical Nutrition* in 2003, had already found that living as a vegetarian for seventeen years would extend your life span by 3.6 years.[59] Still, it can be very comforting (and motivating) to know what our chromosomes are up to when we're feeding them all this yummy food.

So what do you think: How will you spend your extra time on this big beautiful planet? Mother Nature is kicking out all this bounty to make sure we can stick around a little longer—the least we can do is take her up on the offer, and help her out in the process.

chapter 3

OMD for the Planet

A first draft of this book started with a detailed look at climate change, until I realized that half my family would put the book down immediately and use it as a doorstop. For many people, climate change is either too overwhelming or too depressing, or maybe (like many of my family members) you're not entirely convinced that climate change is even a thing. And a whole lot of people are worrying about their day-to-day survival—paying bills, keeping their jobs, finding good childcare or taking care of a sick relative—to think about a warming planet.

Climate change can also be a colossal snoozefest. When we hear about it, we tune out. We numb out. We change the channel. There are only so many times you can hear about the worst fires on record, the worst hurricane season, the worst droughts, floods, heat waves . . .

Part of this, I think, is our tendency to shut down when things are overwhelming. We hear the statistics on the news and how dire the situation sounds—yet we look outside, see the sun shining, hear the birds chirping, and it just doesn't seem *that bad*.

We should probably be a tiny bit grateful for our capacity for denial. Our brains have evolved to allow us a certain amount of healthy dissociation when faced with enormous problems we *think* we can't solve. Not absorbing the enormity of the danger facing us probably makes it a lot easier for us to get through our average week without curling up in the fetal position and never leaving the house.

That's the good part.

The bad part of denial is that it can stop us from evolving, expanding our minds, and employing our imaginations to create real solutions. In the case of climate change, that would be a pity— because this enormous, catastrophic, potentially world-destroying problem is one that we *can* solve. And we could start in the next five minutes, with OMD.

Our Plates, Our Planet

I'll never forget when I first "saw" the true impact of animal agriculture, and how central it was to so many environmental challenges we were facing. I was attending what felt like my ninetieth meeting about climate change at an environmental NGO, watching yet another gut-wrenching presentation on the devastations around the globe. As a member of their leadership council, I had attended these meetings every month for almost ten years. So many terrifying statistics, and so few solutions. After each of these sessions, I would drive home completely depressed.

But on this particular day, Jim and I had already taken that memorable walk on the beach, the walk where we first started to see the glimmer of hope and possibility in reversing climate change through a plant-based lifestyle. I was already starting to think about animal agriculture's impact on the earth. And as I watched slide after slide showing all these horrors—deforestation, ocean acidification, habitat loss, rising temperatures and sea levels, shrinking ice caps—in my mind's eye, I suddenly visualized a flower with all these environmental issues on its petals, and "animal agriculture" at the center—what I now call the "OMD flower."

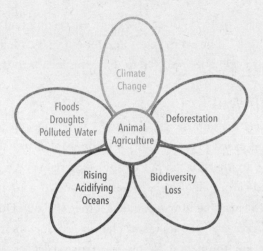

Since our family had gone plant-based, I'd become obsessed with how animal agriculture was hurting the planet. I'd learned that animal agriculture produced runoff that polluted rivers, lakes, and oceans and was a leading driver of algal blooms and dead zones in large bodies of water. Animal agriculture was a leading cause of land use change—all that land needed for livestock and the feed for livestock—which is a primary cause of extinction. Animal agriculture also produced some of the most damaging greenhouse gases, including a huge percentage of methane emissions, and that methane might be as much as thirty-four times more damaging than CO_2.[1,2] Yow!

The OMD flower brought all this together for me, giving me a beautiful, succinct image of the simple, elegant solution. I thought, *What I choose to eat to reduce inflammation can also help feed the bees and save the wolves. . . . What I eat to protect my heart can also revitalize the dead zones in the oceans. . . . What I eat to fight off osteoporosis can also save water. . . . What I eat to prevent cancer can also reduce greenhouse gas emissions. . . . What I eat to give myself more energy can also help regrow the forests. . . .*

The image of that flower was more energizing and optimistic than anything I'd heard in that room for ten years. I left the meeting that day even more resolved to share this idea with the world.

Win-Win-Win

In our quest for knowledge, Jim and I were eager to learn more from plant-based experts, and we really wanted to help them to talk to one another. In the fall of 2013, we organized a summit of plant-based-eating advocates, to get everyone in a room together and brainstorm about how we could get the word out. Our goal was to bring together all the rock-star plant-based doctors in the same room with environmental NGOs and thought leaders. They each had their own audience—but were they talking to one another and did they understand their common mission? We wanted them to realize the point of connection and link between sustainable eating, health, and the planet.

Renowned plant-based health authors and advocates Dean Ornish, Caldwell and Rip Esselstyn, Colin and Nelson Campbell, and John and Mary McDougall were there. And representing the environment, *Food Choice and Sustainability* author Richard Oppenlander, *Diet for a New America* author John Robbins, businessman/philanthropist Craig McCaw, *The Climate Wars* author Eric Pooley, creator of the Process Communication Model Taibi Kahler—and others—all participated in our roundtable discussion, mostly centered around health.

It quickly became clear that whether we were concerned about health, the environment, or animal cruelty, we all had the same goal and mission: to reduce meat and dairy production and consumption. Each had their own inspiration for choosing to eat this way, all valid in and of themselves. Each could have created their own flower diagram, with their own reasons to avoid animal products. But it didn't matter whether you went plant-based for environmental or ethical or health or financial or social justice reasons. Any one of those reasons, any one of those motivations, would have the same result: plant-based eating would help the earth.

Plant-based eating was an absolute win-win-win!

Spreading the word, improving access to and education about, and—most important—helping everyone fall in love with plant-based eating was now what I was meant to do for the rest of my life. Faced with so many unfathomably gigantic, seemingly unsolvable problems, we could all, every one of us, have a quantifiable, observable, positive impact. Simply by eating more plants, we could all make a difference—today!—and I couldn't wait to get started right away.

That was over six years ago, and I have never looked back. In the years since, I've convinced so many different people, from all walks of life—hundreds of little kids, family members, friends, work colleagues, Texas ranchers, New Zealand dairy farmers (as well as the governor general and her husband), actors, teachers, directors, titans of industry, Navy SEALS—even proudly carnivorous, professional-sister-teasing older brothers from Oklahoma—how powerful eating just one meal a day for the planet can be.

No joke: If everyone cuts down a little bit on their meat consumption, we could reduce global food-related emissions by one-third by 2050; if we go vegetarian, we can cut it by almost two-thirds.[3] That kind of shift will help get us a good way toward achieving our emission reduction goals from the Paris Agreement, the benchmarks scientists have said we need to reach by 2050 in order to slow the warming of the planet. (And even if our elected leaders opt out of the Agreement, we can still choose to be a part of it. We Are Still In [WASI] is a US coalition committed to facing climate change and includes 2,500 leaders, from mayors to governors, college presidents to CEOs, representing 127 million Americans and $6.2 trillion—and we are definitely in this together.)

That emission reduction could happen even before we start

talking solar- and wind-power industries, or electric cars becoming the norm, or even whatever amazing thing the scientists and engineers will develop by then. That's just from what we put on our plates for dinner.

And on the deadly serious flip side? If we don't address animal agriculture in some way, and if we in higher income countries allow our extremely high intake to carry on unabated as low- and middle-income countries consumption continues to rise, experts say we might not have a chance of meeting the Paris Agreement goals.[4] Simply put: We can't meet our climate goals if we don't collectively change our diet.[5]

WHAT DOES CLIMATE CHANGE LOOK LIKE WHERE YOU LIVE?

While polar ice caps melting can seem so far away, many of us already see the signs of climate change right in our own neighborhoods. Some signs have been increasing, slowly but surely, for years. Less (or more) snow than you had when you were a kid. More triple-digit-temperature days than ever before. Shorter winters, longer summers. Prolonged, multiyear drought. Drenching rains that start to overpower gutters and sewers. More and more local flooding. More and more friends being diagnosed with Lyme disease. Mudslides—terrifying ones.

When we used to talk about "global warming," people would point outside at snow on the ground, and say, "Still snowy here"—disregarding the general trend of temperatures around the globe. Now we call it "climate change," but the signs we see in our day-to-day lives are probably more accurately called "global weirding"—the earth's energy balance has changed and the weather and other atmospheric patterns are so off-kilter, so different from the way they were just ten or twenty years ago.

Have you noticed any of these signs in your area of the States?

Northeast: More drenching rain, heat waves, fish die-off

Southeast: More intense tropical storms and hurricanes, intense flooding, extreme heat

Midwest: More flooding, extreme heat

Great Plains: Increased competition for water

Southwest: More intense temperatures, drought, insect outbreaks, wildfires, reduced water supply and agricultural yields

Northwest: Coastal erosion, sea level rise, increased ocean acidity, wildfires, insect outbreaks, tree diseases

Alaska: Sea ice receding, glaciers shrinking, thawing permafrost, wildfires (Alaska has warmed twice as fast as the rest of the country)

Hawai'i: Increased coral bleaching, disease outbreak, possible increased tropical storms, coastal erosion from sea level rise[6]

Think about your town or the place where you grew up—how has the weather pattern shifted since you were a kid? How about where you live now—what are the changes you see all around you?

We're seeing these signs all over the world:[7]

Europe: More intense temperatures, intense rainfall, shifting animal migration patterns, more drought

Africa: More intense flooding, more severe drought, reduction in crop yields, intense risk of heat-related mortality, reduction in air quality

South America: Sea level rise, land degradation and desertification, glacial melt, intense risk of heat-related mortality, changing water availability

Australia: Heightened pressure on water supply, bush fires, rising sea levels, ocean acidification, bleaching and impending death of coral reefs, loss of habitat

Asia: More intense and frequent storms, devastating
   flooding, sea level rise, more drought, increased risk
   of heat-related mortality and water- and vector-borne
   diseases, reduction in air quality
Instead of getting distraught, we can take action—just one
meal a day can help reverse this pattern, and save our Earth.

OMD: The Simple, Elegant Solution

To truly understand everything that's going on in climate change science, you would need to have a working knowledge of atmospheric chemistry, oceanography, biology, hydrology, glaciology, biogeochemistry, paleoclimatology . . . and some people truly do like to geek out on that stuff. For most of us, that kind of info makes us shut down or bores us to tears. We feel depressed, powerless.

That's where my new, plant-based OMD flower image came in for me. In one glance, it helped me see everything really simply. But rather than dwell on the doom-and-gloom version of this image, I then flipped it, and placed plant-based agriculture where it belongs: in the center of everything. Let's talk about each petal of the OMD flower image and how it intersects with plant-based eating at its center.

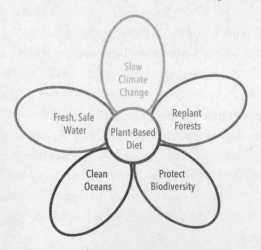

Slow Climate Change

Climate change is perhaps the biggest single challenge we face and affects all others, threatening our very survival as a species. And it's directly tied to animal agriculture and the impact our farming practices have on the earth. As Jonathan Foley of California Academy of Sciences puts it, "Without a doubt, agriculture is the single most powerful force unleashed on this planet since the end of the Ice Age—and it rivals climate change—and they're both happening at the same time."

Sometimes I wonder if we'd absorb the urgency of what faces us a little bit more if we all were a little bit closer to the critically impacted zones. I think that's why our visit to the tiny Micronesian atoll Ulithi, in the days before Jim did his Challenger Deep dive, has stayed with me for so long.

Jim is an avid diver and incredibly passionate about the earth and ocean health. In 2012 he mounted the *DEEPSEA CHALLENGE* Expedition to advance ocean science and explore the deep marine trench systems in the Western Pacific, culminating in a historic, solo descent to the Challenger Deep, the deepest place on the planet. Jim had spent seven years working with a team of scientists, designing and co-engineering the revolutionary *DEEPSEA CHALLENGER* submersible and science platform (which is still the deepest-diving manned marine vehicle in the world). I was there when Jim descended into the ocean depths, diving 35,756 feet into the Challenger Deep, almost 7,000 feet deeper than Mount Everest is high. I wouldn't have wanted to be anywhere else.

Jim's dive was big news in that corner of the world, as he and his team had done significant exploration and test dives in the area in preparation for the historic event. Ulithi, just 180 miles from the Mariana Trench, was the ancestral home to a master navigator, someone who learned the traditional science of using nature (the stars and seas, clouds and wind) as a compass on long ocean crossings. The people of Ulithi wanted to bless Jim's voyage in a special ceremony that hadn't been performed in years. The tribal elders anointed him with turmeric oil, and they put a headdress and a sarong on him as part of the ritual. There was singing and chanting. The whole experience was so moving. It was a tremendous honor for Jim.

The only way onto the island was by invitation and offer of a gift. The community had requested rice, so we brought many 500-kilogram bags. While we were there, I toured the local school and talked to the teachers, and learned that the island used to be fully independent. They had long fished from the ocean, grown and eaten taro, and collected coconuts and other island fruits. But even back in 2012, the people of Ulithi were already feeling the effects of rising sea levels; they could only grow 50 percent of the taro they had once been able to grow because their lands had become brackish. The seawater was seeping into their soil. This was the reason they wanted rice.

If we don't reverse climate change, Ulithi will likely have to relocate its entire community to survive. Think of it: For an ancient seafaring, island culture—a culture that was once proudly independent and sustainable—abandoning their islands may be just a few decades away. And while their situation is more immediately dire, our waterfront cities and communities are just as vulnerable. Experts believe the sea levels could rise between one and five feet—in some places, even more—by the end of the century, and no coastal area in the world will be safe.[8] According to *National Geographic*, by 2100, about 670 towns and cities along the coastline of mainland United States will face flooding on a monthly basis—everywhere from the Boston area to Miami to Oakland, California, even four out of five New York boroughs, will be chronically under water.[9,10]

How is change happening so quickly? Methane, carbon dioxide, and other greenhouse gas emissions are warming the planet. You may immediately picture a factory spewing smoke into the skyline or the exhaust from your car, but would you believe that a major contributor is our addiction to beef and dairy? Cows emit crazy amounts of methane, which the EPA estimates will be thirty-four times more damaging than carbon dioxide over a hundred-year time period.[11] And the production of beef generates six times more greenhouse gases (including carbon dioxide, methane, and nitrous oxide) than the production of chicken, and up to 45 times more than the production of soy products (by calorie).[12] Cows alone produce over 65 percent of the emissions of the entire animal agriculture industry—over 40 percent from beef and 20 percent from dairy.[13] Combined, all activities involved in producing livestock worldwide produce 14.5 percent of global greenhouse gas emissions, according to the United Nations Food and Agriculture Organization—whose model and research is supported by the scientific community.[14,15]

Here's the bottom line: that's more emissions than the entire transportation sector combined. Take every boat, ship, plane, train, automobile, motorcycle, moped, monorail, you name it—add all their emissions from burning fossil fuels together—and meat and dairy still beat it. The World Meteorological Organization measured more carbon dioxide in the atmosphere at the end of 2016 than at any time in the prior eight hundred thousand years.[16]

Those emissions are melting the ice caps. According to NASA, the sea ice of the Arctic has shrunk about 13 percent every decade since 1979.[17] And then there are these methane hydrates, massive natural reservoirs of methane currently trapped deep under permafrost and the ocean floor. If those ice caps melt, or those ocean floor reserves are destabilized by warming, all that incredibly potent methane will be released, which will rapidly speed up climate change—possibly past the point of no return.

And, of course, as the ice caps melt, the sea levels will rise. They've already risen almost ten inches since the start of the twentieth century.[18] We hear "rising sea level" on the news, we watch disaster movies, we try to imagine what will happen—but the people of Ulithi are truly *living it*, every day. That water is rising, and they are watching it rise. Their home and way of life, their entire world, will soon be swallowed up and wiped out—the first of many similar events to come.

It is all connected to animal agriculture. This is why OMD is so powerful—over the course of one year, one person's OMD keeps 772 pounds of carbon emissions out of the atmosphere—the equivalent of keeping a car completely off the road for almost a month.

Replant the Forests

In 2010, Jim was invited to speak at the Manaus Conference on Global Sustainability alongside Al Gore and other noted environmentalists. One was Atossa Soltani, from the organization Amazon Watch, whom we'd met at a Global Green event the year before. She told us about the Brazilian government's plan to build the Belo Monte hydroelectric dam, which, when built, would dam up some fifty miles of the Xingu River, a principal tributary of the Amazon, decimate the indigenous cultures that have depended on it for millennia, and devastate the rain forest. And Belo Monte is only one of sixty hydroelectric dams planned in the Amazon Basin in the next few decades, to meet the continent's surging electric energy demands.

What we heard appalled us. This was a real-life *Avatar*, an energy battleground like too many around the world affecting indigenous peoples, upending their traditional cultures and destroying their lands.

After a brief first visit, we returned to Brazil a month later, journeying far up the Xingu River to a remote Kayapo village. A warrior people, as well as great orators, the Kayapo were working hard to organize their fellow indigenous tribes for a massive show of resistance in Brasília, Brazil's capital city. We came to lend our voice.

On the way out of the Kayapo village, we flew over hundreds of miles of rain forest thinking, *How could all this ever be destroyed?* only to see it stop abruptly, replaced by cattle ranches and farmland for feed. Then we flew on for hours across this devastated landscape. Gone were the verdant green "lungs of the world," replaced with tens of thousands of acres of feedlot. Cows gobble up twenty-eight times more land for every ton of meat produced than even pork, chicken, or eggs—which, in turn, consume up to six times more resources than potatoes, wheat, or rice.[19] Eighty percent of global deforestation is driven by agriculture—and this rate climbs to ninety percent in Latin America.[20,21] In Brazil, animal agriculture—to meet the rising international demand for beef—is responsible for 80 percent of all Amazon rain forest loss. About 450,000 square kilometers of Brazilian rain forest have been cleared for cattle ranching.[22]

During our first two trips, our guides pointed out the encroachment into the rain forest of soy and corn fields, feed crops for the cattle. But it wasn't until two years later, when I was sitting in that meeting at the environmental NGO, that I suddenly *got it*. The moment I saw the flower diagram in my head, all those images came flooding back—the brutal scars those industrial farms had ripped through the middle of the rain forest. This is why steering clear of beef and dairy on OMD has the biggest impact: every quarter-pound hamburger we don't eat saves 318 square feet of rainforest. (Learn more in "Your Burger x 50 Billion Served," page 78.)

Protect Biodiversity

Ironically, the estimated fifty-six billion animals raised for food each year are also one of the leading causes of animal extinction—and if current trends continue, that livestock inventory is expected to double by 2050.[23] The enormous amount of land needed to raise and grow feed for livestock results in land use change, as well as habitat loss, which leads to devastating biodiversity loss.

My daughter Claire has always loved wolves. At MUSE, every child is encouraged to develop their research interest or passion, which they can then study in whatever way speaks to them. For four years, Claire's passion was wolves, and every year, she got deeper and deeper into the subject. At one point, she showed me a video on YouTube about how wolves, once hunted out of existence at Yellowstone National Park, were finally reintroduced into the park after seventy years—and how their reintroduction revitalized the entire ecosystem. (Check out the video about trophic cascades called "How Wolves Change Rivers" on YouTube to get a sense of their impact.[24])

Given the wolves' importance to the ecosystem, you may be wondering, *Why were they driven out to begin with?* To protect the beef cattle on the surrounding farms. The wolves' eradication had caused an environmental collapse inside the park—all for that almighty burger. The wolves are one clear example of why animal agriculture is one of the leading drivers of biodiversity loss and species extinction. Not only does animal agriculture drive the wholesale conversion of natural lands and forests to farmland—around 30 percent of the world's land surface is now used to rear animals[25]—but conflict between those raising livestock and wildlife has led to the systematic extermination of important carnivore species around the world.[26] A study has also found that 30 percent of biodiversity loss on land is linked to animal agriculture.[27] Because beef uses twenty times more land per gram of protein than do legumes,[28] its resource needs gobble up forests and overtake grasslands, diminishing and denuding ecosystems for native plants and animals. In their place is planted pesticide- and fertilizer-intensive monoculture crops such as corn and soybeans.[29] Tragically, every day, we lose upwards of 80,000 acres of tropical rainforest—taking with them 135 plant, animal, and insect species. *Every day.* That's *50,000* species every year.[30]

OMD can help. By cutting our own intake by one-third, we'll

begin to reduce demand. Cattle are expensive to raise, so if people aren't buying beef, smart livestock farmers will likely find another crop to raise, like pulses or other plant proteins. That faltering trend line will discourage new suppliers from investing in livestock. We've already seen the first glimmers of this dynamic at work in the dairy industry, where reduced consumer demand for milk is starting to drive smart dairy farmers into plant-based milks instead. (See "If We Lower Demand, We Can Lower Production" on page 81 for more.)

Clean Oceans

Around the world, we see yet more floods, more algal blooms, more loss of coastline and animal habitats. Dead zones form in both fresh- and saltwater systems when runoff from fertilizers sprayed on corn and soy crops drains into the water, causing overgrowth of algae, which then chokes off the oxygen supply to the native plant and animal life in the water. The water becomes hypoxic, with such low oxygen concentration that the plants and animals within it suffocate and die, or migrate to other areas.

According to a 2008 study in the journal *Science*, the size and number of dead zones around the world has grown exponentially since the 1960s.[31] When that study was published a decade ago, scientists had identified dead zones in more than four hundred systems, covering more than 245,000 square kilometers—and the issue is only escalating. When it was measured in August 2017, the Gulf of Mexico had a dead zone the size of New Jersey—and it had recently grown to about 40 percent larger than its average size over the prior five years.[32]

Once again, halting animal agriculture could be a big part of the solution. A dead zone in the northern Black Sea had been growing since the 1960s, but after the collapse of the Soviet Union in 1989 and the ensuing economic collapse in Central and Eastern Europe, fertilizer use and livestock farming in the Danube River watershed was sharply decreased. In just a few years, by the mid-1990s, the size of the Black Sea dead zone was dramatically reduced, and by 2007 had been virtually eliminated.[33]

We don't have to wait for an economic collapse to create change. Simply reducing the amount of meat and dairy we collectively eat will directly reduce harmful fertilizer and animal waste runoff, which will allow the dead zones and aquatic ecosystems to rebound. Our choices absolutely *can* make a difference.

Conserve Fresh Water

The production of meat both requires and pollutes large amounts of water. Almost a third of the freshwater used in agriculture goes toward raising animals. On top of the water needed to grow the feed, water is also used for the animals' drinking water, in preparing their food, and in maintaining the farm. For example, each quarter-pound cheeseburger sucks up 1,800 *gallons* of water before it hits your belly. (That's twenty-five bathtubs full of precious water—just for one hamburger!) But beef is hardly the only water-waster in animal products. Every egg requires forty-three gallons, as does a cup of milk. (Think of that: 1 cup of milk requires 688 cups of water to produce.)

Think that's nuts? A single *tablespoon* of butter takes almost twenty-two gallons of water to produce.

Now imagine that milk concentrated into cheese, and that becomes seventy-five *gallons* for a single two-ounce serving. Seventy-five gallons of clean water reduced to a tiny cube of cheese on the end of a toothpick at a cocktail party. That's the same as turning your shower on full blast and just walking away—for a half hour. For a tiny cube of cheese.

Now consider what an immediate impact your OMD makes on your water footprint. While plant foods do require *some* water to be grown, the difference is just staggering. Swapping out one pound of real beef for a pound of "beefy" crumbles in that pot of chili will save you 1,733 gallons of water. For the same fifteen grams of protein you would get in a single hamburger patty, you could add three tablespoons of pea protein powder into a yummy smoothie—and save 567 gallons of water in one glass.

Imagine Your Impact

Nobody wakes up thinking, "Boy, I really want to destroy the planet, pollute our waterways, make our oceans sick, or cut down a forest today." Of course not. Most of us have good intentions—we just have no idea where to start or any idea that our food choices contribute to climate change. I didn't!

Climate change was largely created by decisions made by people far in the past, far beyond our control. But what also got us here was a slow and steady accumulation of many individual choices, made on a day-by-day basis: Spraying pesticides on our weeds instead of yanking them out by hand. Driving the SUV instead of the compact car. Choosing plastic instead of paper. Buying a bottle of water instead of using the water fountain. Eating meat and/or dairy at every meal. Or just consuming tons of stuff in general.

These individual choices have accumulated and have now become bigger issues. But that same exact principle—the repetition of small daily choices—now affords us our absolute *best* chance of turning things around. If everyone can start to make one slightly different choice, once a day, we can have a huge impact.

A study by the University of Oxford found that, every day, most meat eaters in the United Kingdom generate about sixteen pounds of CO_2 from their diets, while vegetarians and fish eaters generate about eight pounds. Fully plant-based eaters produce a little over six pounds—60 percent less than typical meat eaters.[34] So with your first OMD, you've already cut almost 20 percent of your total personal carbon and water footprint for the day. BAM! That easy. All before you turn the thermostat down or switch to a wind-power electric company or bring along a reusable water bottle. Eating plant-based is like putting all your good environmental citizenship choices on steroids.

Your Burger x 50 Billion Served

When we talk about an individual's potential impact with OMD, burgers are a great place to start. Burgers became the original and most favored fast food for a reason: you can hold an entire meal in one hand while you're driving down the freeway. Right now, as a country, Americans eat an average of three burgers per person a week. An eye-popping fifty billion every year. Every single one of those cheeseburgers requires 1,800 gallons of water to produce. And each burger is the equivalent of driving almost fifteen miles in an exhaust-spewing car.[35]

Now consider that, worldwide, we already have almost 7.5 billion mouths to feed. We add seventy-five million more people (about the population of Germany) to the earth every year. We're projected to hit 9.7 billion by the year 2050.

Every one of those mouths will require thousands of calories a day to survive. Now consider that the resources needed to feed one or two people a meat-based diet could hypothetically feed ten people a plant-based diet.[36] Or, if we strip this argument down to its essentials: Every time you opt for the veggie burger instead of the beef burger, you're (hypothetically) feeding nine hungry people who would otherwise go without.

Suddenly, our choice for this one humble sandwich gives us an incredible climate-protecting, resource-saving, and extra-people-feeding opportunity—one that compounds itself daily.

Now, let's say you and your partner or friend skip that eight ounces of beef *once a week* for a year. By the end of that year, you'll have saved:

904 miles of driving

¾ acre of land

48,100 gallons of water being guzzled up by that sweet cow (That's not a typo—impressive, right?)

Then let's say you both skip that same eight ounces of beef *once a day* for a year. At the end of that year, you'll have saved:

6,345 miles (the equivalent of driving from Portland, Maine, to San Diego—and back!)

5.3 acres of land (over four football fields)

337,100 gallons of water (half the water in an Olympic-size pool)

Bear in mind—this is just you and your partner or friend, going without beef, for *one meal a day*. I'm not even counting the other animal products in your meal: the butter on your potato, or the milk in your glass, or the ranch dressing on your salad.

Isn't that just the coolest thing ever?

Now, let's say we can get everyone in your family of four to do this. Keep it simple and say you average about one pound of meat per family dinner. So you guys all get together and decide this OMD thing is no biggie, and you can easily skip that one serving of meat every day.

At the end of year one, just giving up that *one serving of meat a day*, your family will have saved:

12,690 miles (driving from San Francisco to New York—the scenic route!—*four times*)

10.5 acres of land (over eight football fields)

675,250 gallons of water (the amount needed to fill that Olympic-size pool)

And the resources your family will have saved could hypothetically feed an extra 13,140 hungry people a nourishing plant-based meal.

Again, this is from *one serving of meat a day*. That's it. Just skipping the steak. Or maybe eating vegetarian chili instead of chili con carne. Or just having bean burritos instead of beef burritos.

If every family in America did this, we could—with this one act alone—help change the course of our future. Can you see why I am so excited about this!? How much potential we have to make a difference? How much impact even the very smallest change can have?

Now, think back to those overwhelming stories you see on TV—the visions of drought, and hurricanes, climate refugees, crops drying up, whole neighborhoods of houses destroyed by tropical storms or wildfires, whole islands disappearing under the waves . . .

And now think of how insurmountable it seems to be to get public officials to even recognize climate change, let alone do something about it. How they've withdrawn support from the agencies that protect our air, rivers and lakes, and land from pollution. (Who woulda thought clean air and water for our kids was political?)

If it's personally possible for us to make this big of a difference, to take such huge strides to save our planet, with such a tiny shift . . . isn't it exciting to imagine joining together to make an enormous, collective impact?

When we are long gone, our grown children may one day look around and wonder why we didn't do everything possible to reverse the course we're on. That thought, that image, haunts me. I can't live with that . . . can you? We are accountable to them, and every generation that comes after them. And now that I've been sitting with all of this for a while, it's just gotten so hard for me to imagine any burger worth that feeling.

If We Lower Demand, We Can Lower Production

For better or worse, Americans lead the world in food trends. As other developing countries grow more prosperous, many are increasing their meat consumption. Others have been industrialized for decades and have simply been following our lead, increasing their meat consumption by five or ten, even fifteen times, in the past forty years.[37] (And, sadly, they've developed epic levels of obesity and chronic disease at the same pace.) Thankfully, the largest of these countries—China—has recognized the outsize role animal agriculture has in climate change and ill health, and they're taking steps to counter it. Their latest dietary guidelines recommended a *50 percent reduction of meat and dairy* from the current average diet—the equivalent of taking ninety-three million cars off the road.[38]

In contrast, in the United States, there's a political machine in place that's designed to keep us buying and eating more burgers and gallons of milk. Subsidies. Lobbyists. School lunches. Restaurant menus. Procurement practices. The US meat and dairy industries alone spend billions of dollars every year promoting their goods, including sending millions to lobby legislators. Animal agriculture companies (and the grain companies that supply them) get massive subsidies, all of which are paid for with our tax dollars.

So what do we get?

Meat lover's double-stuffed-crust pizza for five dollars. "Got Milk?" campaigns. Mandatory milk servings in public school lunches. The meat and dairy lobby spends serious money to influence us to buy the burger from McDonald's and the quadruple cheese pizza at Pizza Hut. With those cash-for-cows subsidies in place, animal ag companies *over*produce their goods. For example, in 2016, dairy farmers had a "glut" of milk and had to pour out forty-three million gallons—enough to fill sixty-six Olympic-size swimming pools. Then the

USDA swooped in to buy up $20 million of excess cheddar cheese, which it said it would redirect toward food banks and food assistance. The dairy industry also works behind the scenes with the government and other food companies to wiggle that surplus into already dairy-laden products, such as putting more butter into an Egg McMuffin or more cheese on a Taco Bell taco. Think of all those ads for triple cheese pizzas, cheese-filled crusts, and queso-everything—if there's a way government-sponsored marketing group Dairy Management Inc. can shove more cheese onto or into or between a product, they will find it![39,40]

And advertising meat and dairy is big business.

In 2011, McDonald's spent $1.37 billion on advertising, about the same as General Motors, Google, or Apple.[41] When someone says "beef," chances are you reflexively think, *It's what's for dinner*—because the National Cattlemen's Beef Association spent $42 million to make sure of it.[42,43] In 2013 alone—gearing up for a major election year—the meat industry contributed $17.5 million to federal candidates, a courtesy that's been proven to yield tremendous favors when it comes to writing policy.[44]

Ever wonder why the salad at McDonald's is seven bucks, and the burger is a dollar? What is the true cost? And who is paying it?

In the meantime, McDonald's is testing out the "McVegan" burger in Finland and Sweden. In the UK, ever since the mad cow disease crisis of the late eighties and nineties, McDonald's serves the Vegetable Deluxe, a patty made with chickpeas and spiced with coriander and cumin.

This all adds up to a lot of consumption. Per capita, Americans now eat a staggering 180 pounds of meat a year.[45] As Raj Patel, a research professor at the LBJ School of Public Affairs at the University of Texas at Austin and author of *Stuffed and Starved*, has said, "If the world were to eat as much meat as the United States does, we'd need at least four more planets."

We just don't need all this animal protein—all available data tell us this level of consumption is making us sick. We eat way more protein than our bodies can even use—and it doesn't even have to be protein in the first place. The first best thing we can do to make a large-scale impact on the health of our people and our environment is to create less demand for meat and dairy.

The best way to do this? Change the way you shop, order, and eat. With every dollar we spend on our food, we are letting the industry know, "Hey, keep doing what you're doing. More, please." Every dollar that we spend on a cheap burger or a roast beef sandwich or a steak tells the industry we want to continue to contribute to biodiversity loss, extinction, factory farming, and environmental degradation. But reduced demand diminishes output.

That moment of sitting down to a meal is a point of such opportunity, both for awareness of our connection to the earth and for actual power to change its future. In critical, black-and-white, dollars-and-cents influence, we can have a direct, positive, long-lasting impact on the environment by forgoing that cheeseburger and having a delicious meal of BBQ "Chicken" Sliders with Classic Coleslaw (page 236) or The King's Shepherd's Pie (page 241) instead.

Every time you choose a chicken breast over a beef burger, every time you choose a veggie burger over a chicken breast, you're doing something downright revolutionary: You are telling the corporations of the world, Big Ag, the lobbyists, the government, that they must change. That the meat and dairy industries aren't as powerful as they think they are. That they can't control policy. That they can't go down to Brazil and mow down another acre of rain forest in your name. That they can't keep clean water away from people in Flint, Michigan, and give it to cows in Oklahoma in your name.

And believe me, the meat and dairy industries are listening. Dairy milk consumption dropped by over 20 percent between 2000 and 2016,[46] and almost half of all Americans now drink alternative, nondairy milks.[47] As a result of this decreased consumer demand, Elmhurst Dairy, in Queens, New York, stopped producing dairy milk after ninety years and shifted their production to a range of plant-based milks. In 2016 Tyson Foods, one of the largest producers of chicken, beef, and pork in the country, quietly became a 5 percent shareholder of Beyond Meat, a company that has developed plant-based meat analogues that are dead ringers for the real thing.[48] (And then acquired even more stock the next year.[49]) Animal agriculture companies are beginning to see where this is headed. We consumers hold the ultimate power—the power of the purse—and we can use it to send a strong message and speed the evolution of plant-based foods.

Imagine what would happen if more of us ate meat and dairy less often. Many of those industrial farms would be forced to find other crops. Because other farmers wouldn't have to produce animal feed, some of those fields could be diversified to meet the demand of all these new plant-based eaters who like a little variety on their plates. Instead of just corn and soy and alfalfa, we could have chickpeas and lentils and peas. Instead of needing to expend ten calories of resources to produce one calorie of beef, we could skip the cow and just feed ten people. Stimulated by the demand for that rainbow of plant-based food, biodiversity would start to come back to the land, bringing back missing forms of wildlife, giving local farmers richer soil and healthier workers . . . and the virtuous cycle could continue indefinitely. By supporting more ecological methods of farming, we could directly drive a change in our agricultural landscape and create an opportunity to let nature back in—thereby reversing this huge loss of the wildlife killed during the clearing of farmlands in the twentieth century.

True change, lasting change, doesn't come from the leadership down. Leadership only changes when the people wake up and demand that change. Think of it: We can influence *them*—the corporations, the lobbyists, the politicians. We can protect the climate, we can preserve the clean air, clean water, the rain forests. Just by what we put on our plate. As Dr. Vandana Shiva says, "If governments won't solve the climate, hunger, health, and democracy crisis, then the people will."

That is how change happens. *That* is how we can save the environment. Doing OMD, eating plant-based, is a win-win-win—it truly doesn't matter if you do it for your health, the animals, or the environment—every living thing on earth wins.

Your Next Bite Can Start to Make a Difference

One night last summer, the kids and I prepared a green feast. My eldest, Jasper, and his wife, Solimar ("Soli"), were visiting, en route to their home in New Zealand after a visit to her family in Guatemala. They gathered greens from the garden to make a big herbal salad. Soli made a Peruvian salad with avocado, olive oil, salt, and pepper. My youngest daughter, Rose, made her pasta with fresh herbs. Quinn made his delicious pesto. We put out tons of hummus and dips, and a bunch of chopped vegetables, to try all the different flavors together. And then we warmed up some leftover plant-based mac and cheese to round it all out.

Watching my kids cook and share food, I felt such fierce love for them. I had a flashback to when I was a little girl in my mom's hometown, Oakdale, Louisiana, and being there with her mom, my grandmother, and my family for our annual summer vacation. That's where we developed our taste for creamed corn and black-eyed peas. On the fifth day or so into our vacation every year, we'd all gather in the kitchen to pull together "snack dinner." We'd pull out the Pickapeppa sauce and pour it over a block of Philadelphia cream cheese and spread it on Ritz crackers. We'd eat smoked oysters and smoked sardines, sliced tomato with mayo and salt and pepper—then we'd just put out all the leftovers from the fridge to fill out the meal.

It felt so good to re-create this in a greener, cleaner version of snack dinner with all my kids. When we have time to do it, these are our favorite kinds of dinners—everyone contributes something, and we all try a bunch of different tastes and combinations. Meals like this feel kind of reverent in a way too. It makes us appreciate all of nature's bounty that's going to make us stronger and healthier and give us energy for another day, and protect the planet while we're at it.

The memory of that meal has stuck with me ever since. Maybe it was all the beautiful colors. Maybe it was Jasper and Soli being here with us, seven thousand miles from their home, and all my kids being together at the same time.

Our sacred family time is Sunday dinner. If something gets in the way of this weekly tradition, Jim and I always get an earful from the kids. We all love this ritual.

I love that OMD is, at its core, about taking life one meal at a time. Meals are the most primal means of bringing people together. We connect with our families while we eat foods that connect us to the animals, our community, and the earth on a local and global level. Our lives can be so crazy, but with OMD as the organizing principle of my life, I have a simple, elegant solution—a way to focus my thinking and address everything that matters to me.

Our future has always been the sum total of all our moment-to-moment decisions. And in order to realize these wonderful benefits of OMD, we can begin to make really simple, one-step-at-a-time decisions: Ask for nut or oat milk creamer instead of half-and-half. Leave the chicken off the salad, and double up on walnuts and avocado. Reach for an almond butter and jelly instead of a ham sandwich.

When we make these changes easy, they become instinctive and automatic. When we set ourselves up for success, we realize just how tasty, varied, nourishing, and satisfying plant-based eating is—and we rarely get a chance to miss the ho-hum meat. When we finally experience and understand that the food truly is gratifying and satisfying, we start to feel better and healthier, and to experience a deeper sense of connection to the earth with every meal. We develop a soul-level recognition that this meal, this very bite, is about something larger than us all.

Any movement we can make in the direction of this transition takes us closer to a planet that is beautiful, fertile, and lush, instead of hurtling toward one that is dry, brittle, and scorched.

I love this inspiration from Joanna Macy from her book *Coming Back to Life:*[50]

We can choose life. Even as we face global climate disruption . . . we can still act for the sake of a livable world. It is crucial that we know this: we can meet our needs without destroying our life support system. We have the scientific knowledge and the technical means to do that. We have the savvy and the resources to grow sufficient quantities of real, unaltered food. We know how to protect clean air and water. We can generate energy we require through solar power, wind, tides, algae and fungi. We can exercise our moral imagination to bring our lifestyles and consumption into harmony with all living systems of Earth. All we need is the collective will.

By choosing foods that are pure, safe, and clean, we can live in peaceful awareness that we are doing the best for ourselves, our families, and our future. Whether you are a spiritual person or a deeply ethical one, there is so much solace that comes along with "coming correct" on food. When you know you will be able to look back and feel good about your choices, no matter what they are, your moral slate gets pretty darn clean pretty fast.

As a mom, I know how difficult it can be to manage all the different parts of our lives—how to find time to be the best parent, sister, daughter, friend, wife, artist, worker we can be—and still find time for ourselves. I've witnessed that learning how to bring more plant-based eating into your life opens up space to invest in *you*—to learn new cooking techniques, to linger longer in the produce aisle, to experiment with new fruits or vegetables, to ask questions at the farmers' market—while you also give voice to that part of you that sometimes can get drowned out by the daily comings and goings of a busy life.

OMD gives you a format to reengage with your food, to really dig in and feel and experience your food once again, to recognize that every bite you take is packed with molecules of the earth, bits of stardust that get to take up residence in your body for a little while before you send them out into the broader universe once again for another spin around the sun. OMD can help you really key into that cycle and recognize your role as a steward and a host and a vehicle for knowledge for the next generations during our oh-so-short time here on earth.

And hopefully, ten, twenty, thirty, forty years in the future, when it comes time to see where these efforts have brought us, to know that when it really mattered, when the time was *now* and we were asked to make a change or lose everything—you'll know you made the right choice. You chose to protect the world and its future and all living things—just by passing up that cheeseburger.

And it worked.

We might be able to die a little more at peace. When we look back over our lives, we'll see more things we can be proud of. We'll know that what we've done has made a difference.

With plant-based eating at the center of my flower, OMD is the simple, elegant solution that pulls all the facets of my life together. It's a meal-planning technique, an avenue to radiant health, a game that helps kids get excited about saving the planet. It's an invitation to make a difference in collective action with others. With this one shift, I know I can take care of the earth, the animals, the people, *my* people, and myself.

Win-win-win!

TAKE THE PLEDGE

Every year at the start of school at MUSE, we talk about OMD and ask the kids and parents to consider their level of commitment—are they ready to join together with other members of the school community, to make the promise to think about the earth, and to dedicate one meal a day to the planet? How about just a pinky promise? Help yourself and your family internalize this commitment to your health and connection with the earth by following this simple practice that allows you to *live it*, every single day.

OMD Pledge
Together with my family, I will eat One Meal a Day for the Planet—or two, or three.

How Much Do I Want to Save?

 EAT 1 PLANT-BASED MEAL A DAY
Save 194,667 gallons of water and
772 pounds of carbon emissions

 EAT 2 PLANT-BASED MEALS A DAY
Save 389,344 gallons of water and
1,543 pounds of carbon emissions

 EAT 3 PLANT-BASED MEALS A DAY
Save 584,001 gallons of water and
2,315 pounds of carbon emissions

PART TWO

The OMD Way

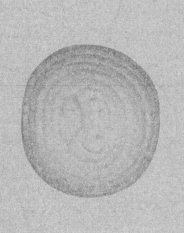

chapter 4

Prepare to OMD

Now, what do you think—are you ready to give it a try?

Remember: It's just one meal a day. OMD. Start small, start right where you are, and plan your first meal. You don't have to overthink it—you can just make a plan, and you'll already be living the OMD way.

Eating more plants is the easiest, least stressful, lowest-maintenance way of making a significant impact in helping to save the world—without spending an extra cent. As Dr. Katz, says, "We can put solar panels on our roof, but we need other people to develop the solar panel technology. We don't need anybody's help to eat more beans and lentils and less beef."

OMD achieves so many objectives simultaneously:

It provides a built-in, daily opportunity to take concrete steps to help fight climate change.

It creates an easy-to-follow framework to increase your and your loved ones' intake of fruits and vegetables.

It cuts intake of inflammatory meat and dairy products by 30 percent.

It reduces your and your family's risk of heart disease, diabetes, and cancer, and begins to extend your life span.

It makes eating well and caring for the earth feasible—and
fun—for the whole family.

It allows you to care for your family, friends, partner, and self,
all at the same time.

My goal with this chapter is to help you realize that, yes, you really
can do this. I am going to make this transition as fun, easy, and delicious as I possibly can.

The beauty of OMD is that you don't have to do a ton of prep, but
I'll share some general guidelines to help you get started right away.
In this chapter, I'll give you all the resources you need to get supplies in the house and prepare, so you can pull off your OMD without a hitch. In chapter 5, "One Meal a Day," I help you get a foothold
and a running start, with more step-by-step guidance to make this
shift for one meal every day. (Inspired to go further? In chapter 6,
"All-In," I explain how to make an overnight transition to plant-
based eating, just like Jim and I did.) In chapter 7, "OMD Recipes,"
I include fail-proof recipes that are sure to please the whole family
and that I guarantee will make it so you don't miss the meat and the
dairy. Many of these recipes come from my kids, my siblings, my
mother or mother-in-love, or my friends. Most are based on dishes
that are typically prepared with meat or dairy. You'll see how easy it
is to make a few swaps so you can still enjoy your favorite meals and
foods in a new, OMD-friendly form.

After a few days on OMD, you may feel different—you likely
won't feel bloated or gassy or *blah* after eating. If you add a few more
plant-based meals, you might feel even lighter, a bit more energized.
Even when you eat a lot, you won't have that post-holiday food
coma. You won't feel hit by a truck. A few more plant-based meals,
and your heart and lungs will pump easier. A few more, and you'll
think clearer and have more mental stamina, and your body will
recover faster after exercise. And if this stuff really sticks with you

and you find you're averaging two or more plant-based meals a day, you'll start to get that "glow" that everyone talks about—your skin gets clearer, softer, smoother, younger-looking. Your body will stop aging so quickly. You will likely lose a couple of years off your face. You will begin to effortlessly manage your weight, easily dropping any extra pounds or automatically maintaining a healthy weight.

As you go along, I would love to hear about your experiences and have you share them with others on the OMD journey. Please come to https://www.facebook.com/OMD4thePlanet/ and share them with us.

Four Factors of OMD Motivation

I know it can be a little difficult knowing where to begin and how to summon up the courage to try something new. I want to help you forget outdated notions that might be holding you back, and give you the info you need to lean into this challenge with your whole heart.

In 2014, the well-respected British think tank Chatham House published an in-depth research paper entitled *Livestock—Climate Change's Forgotten Sector: Global Public Opinion on Meat and Dairy Consumption.*[1] They surveyed over twelve thousand people in twelve countries, and found that most people were open to eating more plant-based meals once they learned about the issues surrounding animal agriculture. They also found that, across cultural lines, people's attitude toward plant-based eating can be shifted once four key factors are taken into account: price, flavor, food safety, and localized environmental concerns. Let's tackle each of these head on.

Flavor

People are initially a bit worried about not liking the flavors of a plant-based diet, but that's actually one of the huge pluses. Once you start to eat more plant food, your palate will begin to expand very quickly.

You'll start to notice subtle differences between those different varieties. You'll derive more pleasure from eating fresh fruits and vegetables. The blunt cooking instrument of animal fat will cease to be as appealing, because you'll start to associate it with feeling sluggish and sleepy. Butter, cream, and cheese will start to seem like the cavemen of cooking ingredients.

When people say things like, "I don't like plant-based food," I always think of that Joey's refusals of Sam-I-Am's offerings in *Green Eggs and Ham*, stubbornly repeating "I do not like green eggs and ham/I do not like them, Sam-I-Am." I want to ask them, "Do you eat salad? Bean burritos? Do you like peanut butter and jelly? Those are plant-based!"

Full disclosure: I know cheese can be hard to kick, for a very good reason—it's more like a drug than a food. Cheese has the highest concentration of casein, a dairy protein that breaks down into casomorphins—aka dairy opiates. Our own breast milk has a version of these to help our babies grow from seven to eighteen pounds; cow's milk has those casomorphins in there to help woo a baby calf into growing from sixty to *six hundred* pounds. Then when you concentrate that milk into yogurt, or even further, into cheese . . . the cheese platter at the holiday party has become a buffet of morphine cubes.

So if you feel addicted to cheese . . . there's a good chance you are. But never fear—OMD is here! OMD can help you break free. Dr. Neal Barnard's book *The Cheese Trap* is a great read for those of us who struggle with dairy addiction. Try to remind yourself that dairy is ultra-inflammatory and has been linked to osteoporosis, diabetes, heart disease, autoimmune conditions, allergies, neurological conditions, even cancer. In *The China Study*, Dr. Campbell shares his extremely compelling experience of revealing a direct correlation between the consumption of casein and liver cancer. Time to say goodbye!

Nuts: Your OMD Secret Weapon

When you're making the OMD transition and weaning yourself off meat at every meal, *don't be afraid of nuts*. You'll see all kinds of nuts used in the recipes in chapter 7. Nuts are truly a wonder food. With their rich and luscious flavor, protein, and super-nutritious fats, nuts are a great stand-in for animal products during the transition. Enjoy them. (But remember, a little goes a long way. It's not the best idea to sit down and eat a pound of nuts.)

In a 2017 study by the team at the Harvard T.H. Chan School of Public Health, published in the *Journal of the American College of Cardiology*, researchers looked at eating records from over two hundred thousand people over thirty-two years and found that overall consumption of nuts is inversely proportional to risk of cardiovascular disease.[2] In other words, the more nuts we eat, the lower our chances of developing these diseases. Compared with people who didn't eat many (or any) nuts, those who ate a serving of peanuts and tree nuts at least five times per week reduced their risk of coronary heart disease by at least 20 percent.

When I first went plant-based, I ate a lot of cashew butter (my brother Charlie fondly refers to it as "crack butter"). I also used to take sunflower seed butter and just eat it with a spoon. I found that my cravings for that level of fat tapered off after a while. If I eat hummus with tahini now, it feels so rich and yummy.

Now is the time to woo your taste buds to plant-based flavors. Eventually your taste buds change, things balance out, and you may start craving fewer fatty things. Nuts are a good transition tool—a gateway drug to the whole-food, plant-based lifestyle. Besides, when you eat the OMD way, you've already automatically reduced the saturated fat-dense animal products that normally drive up the calories—live a little.

Price

When you eat OMD, you've already automatically cut down on the saturated fat–dense animal products that normally drive up the cost of food. But you could eat an extremely healthy and tasty plant-based meal for under two dollars. How? Rice and beans—the world's least expensive meal, and nearly the most nutritious. You can go to a Mexican, Asian, or Indian market and get a fifteen-pound bag of rice and a ten-pound bag of black beans for thirty dollars, and have your protein bases covered for one hundred different meals. Now, I know that depending on where you live and what time of year it is, sometimes fresh organic produce can be a little bit expensive. But if the protein foundation of your meal tops out at 30 cents, you can afford to splurge on some fresh fruit and vegetables to go with it. *Eat Vegan on $4.00 a Day: A Game Plan for the Budget Conscious Cook* by Ellen Jaffe Jones is a good read for thrifty vegans.

And remember: You don't have to buy fresh produce. Yes, organic fresh produce is the best thing. (Top priority is to avoid the Environmental Working Group's Dirty Dozen, the conventional produce with the highest residue of pesticides—find the list, updated yearly, at https://www.ewg.org/foodnews/dirty_dozen_list.php.) Conventional is next best. But using frozen vegetables is a great, convenient option—especially if you live someplace where you can't get fresh fruits and vegetables year-round. (See "Buy It Fresh (When You Can)" on page 127 for more purchase suggestions.)

With all this in mind, what is still, hands-down, the most expensive item in any grocery store? Meat! Even if the product itself doesn't cost that much because there are many subsidies and policies that keep that price tag low, you're still paying for that in many other ways. Americans have been coasting along on meat and dairy subsidies for decades, allowing the earth and the nameless, faceless people who are working or living in the agricultural zones to absorb all the negative side effects of our cheap meat for years. Here's a good rule of thumb: when you look at any piece of meat in the grocery store, multiply the price by about ten times[3]—that's the true cost that's being borne by agricultural communities, industrial cleanup, climate change, the health system, and our tax dollars (for subsidies), but never shows up on the price tag.

Instead of feeding this unhealthy system, take that money straight to the source and buy your produce at a farmers' market or sign up for a CSA (Community Supported Agriculture) share. Your money will go straight into the pocket of the farmer who produced your food—and you'll be getting your fresh food days or weeks before you would've gotten it if you'd purchased it through an industrial chain. (See the produce buying guide on page 131 for tips on how to buy the best produce and keep it freshest longest.) And then make a habit of picking one day in the week to make a big pot of soup to use up all the remaining veggies before they go to waste.

Take OMD to the Market

When you go to a farmers' market, the benefits increase even more. You're putting money directly into your local economy, cutting out the corporate middle person, and helping farmers keep more of the profits from the sales of the foods they grow. You're reducing the amount of fossil fuel needed to get that produce into your hands (because you're buying local) and improving the quality of the air your family breathes by reducing the emissions in your local environment. If you're buying organic, you're keeping chemicals out of the soil, streams, and air—and out of your body. The foods are fresher, with a higher density of phytonutrients, and they have local pollen attached to them, which "teach" your immune system about the surrounding environment and help prevent seasonal allergies. You protect the heritage and the long-term stability of your local farmers, ensuring that they have a dependable revenue stream and can weather the ups and downs–such as flooding, drought, and temperature variations–that are already starting to come with climate change. Talk about a win-win-win.

Safety

A CDC report from 2013 found that while contamination is found in a wide range of food products (animal and vegetable), *fatalities* from food poisoning were more likely to come from animal products.[4] Studies have shown that when plants like spinach or romaine trigger outbreaks of E. coli, animal agriculture is still the cause: manure-based fertilizer tends to be the source of the contamination.[5]

And the risks don't come from just *E. coli*. A March 2017 report from the European Public Health Alliance cites antibiotic resistance "as one of the most pressing challenges facing the world today," and squarely puts the blame on industrial agriculture as one the largest contributors to antibiotic resistance worldwide.[6] (The same report states "unhealthy diet is the single largest risk factor for the entire burden of chronic diseases in Europe," pointing to the high levels of processed meat and red meat as a prime cause.)

While the study from Chatham House (see page 95) found that we tend to expect the government to protect our food supply, with the massive wave of deregulation currently sweeping Washington, maybe it's about time we started paying a bit closer attention. We may want to be looking for alternative ways to protect ourselves from food contamination—starting with minimizing our exposure to foods most likely to do the most harm.

The animal agriculture industry is licking its lips at the thought of lowered regulations. In September 2017, the National Chicken Council requested that the USDA abandon all limits on speed on chicken evisceration lines (where chickens are cut open and their organs are removed). Note: The limit right now stands at 140 birds per minute—clearly, two or three chickens *per second* is way too slow.

And remember that any environmental toxin or heavy metal consumed by an animal stays in its flesh and continues to concentrate over the animal's lifetime. With every bite of meat or sip of dairy, you're taking in every pesticide in that animal's feed, every antibiotic used to fatten her up faster, every infection overlooked by a less-than-vigilant safety inspection—all the dirty conditions that are perpetuated when people cut corners with health and safety screenings. *Be very, very afraid of cheap meat.* You are swallowing those shady tradeoffs with every bite.

On the flip side, there's that whole saving-your-life safety aspect of plant-based eating. According to the CDC, only about one in ten adults get the recommended number of fruits and vegetables per day. When you're eating plant-based meals, unless you're following a fries-and-bread vegan approach, you'll automatically be eating a higher percentage of produce with every bite. Even if organic vegetables seem beyond your budget for now, please know that any nonorganic vegetable or fruit (fresh or frozen) is way healthier than any kind of animal product.

Local Environmental Concerns

A recent Yale University survey of eighteen thousand Americans found that while 70 percent of Americans believe that climate change is happening, only 40 percent believe it will harm them personally. And yet if you walk into any diner in America, I bet you can strike up a conversation about how weird or abnormal the weather has been these last few years—So dry! So wet! So hot! So cold! We see the evidence all around us—we live in it—yet we sometimes struggle to make the visceral connection between climate change and our daily lives, our towns, our homes.

What Does It Take to Make . . .

Every food we eat, every product we buy, has a unique environmental footprint on the earth. Meat exists on a continuum, as do vegetables, fruits, and nuts and seeds. Sometimes you'll see a highly touted article claiming that lettuce has a higher environmental impact than meat. To get the real story, step back and look at the entire life cycle of that food, from the ground to your table. (Remember that to get one beef calorie you need to use ten plant calories. Let's skip the middle animals.) Check out the differences in the feed and water consumption for each of these types of protein:

TO MAKE 100 CALORIES OF . . .	IT TAKES . . .
Beef	3,600 calories of feed
Pork	1,130 calories of feed
Chicken or turkey	880 calories of feed
Egg	630 calories of feed
Milk	590 calories of feed
Broccoli	0 calories of feed

TO MAKE 100 CALORIES OF . . .	IT TAKES . . .
Beef	43.4 gallons of water
Pork	4.9 gallons of water
Milk	4.5 gallons of water
Chicken or turkey	3.8 gallons of water
Eggs	2.8 gallons of water
Broccoli	2.6 gallons of water

TO MAKE 1 GRAM OF PROTEIN OF . . .	IT TAKES . . .
Pork	over 1 gallon of water
Beef	1 gallon of water
Milk	~⅔ gallons of water
Chicken or turkey	~⅔ gallon of water
Eggs	~⅔ gallon of water
Broccoli	~⅓ gallon of water

By buying your produce directly from a local farmer, not only do you get the freshest flavors and support your local economy, you're also contributing to a healthy ecosystem for your surrounding area in so many different ways. Less gas is burned to bring food into your town. Buying plant-based foods in your community supports those farmers and encourages healthy practices with the soil. Even the bees will be happier, with more food to support them as they go on their pollinating journey.

The Green Eater Meter

As you're moving toward a plant-based diet, it can be helpful and motivating to prioritize your decisions based on what can have the largest impact right away. *Any* shift away from meat and dairy toward plant-based proteins can make a tremendous difference— which is why you don't have to be 100 percent vegan to have a huge impact. As Brian Kateman of the Reducetarian Foundation has pointed out, cutting down from two servings of meat to one has just as much impact as going from one serving to none.[7]

The variation on these items can be so vast, we need to turn to the scientists to help us answer some nagging questions: How much good are we really doing when we give up beef versus chicken versus eggs? We've heard that almonds are really water-intensive—what's the story with that? NPR did a story breaking this down, called "How Almonds Became a Scapegoat for California's Drought," as does One Green Planet's story "Smart Dairy Farmers Are Planting Almond Crops Because Even They Know No One Wants Cow's Milk Anymore." The various types of agricultural methods, the diverse needs of the plants and animals themselves, the transport of fresh foods to market— those are all complex "inputs" that can radically shift a food's actual environmental impact. How can you know what's best?

One way: Put it through the Green Eater Meter.

We worked with Dr. Maximino Alfredo Mejia of the Environmental Nutrition group at Andrews University to answer these questions and help us develop the OMD Green Eater Meter. Dr. Mejia has taken dozens of inputs, everything from fuel to feed to water to emissions, and crunched the numbers to get a composite score for the environmental savings for every recipe in the book. We've also calculated how much water you will save, how much land you are sparing from being cleared, and the equivalent of how many cars you took off the street for how many miles, simply by making that meal plant-based instead of made with meat and dairy.

Now, bear in mind that the Green Meter Eater only measures *savings*, so a traditionally plant-based dish, such as salsa or guacamole, would have a baseline Green Eater Meter score of zero. But a dish like Mom Amis's Creamed Corn (page 231), which swaps out cream, milk, and butter, has a Green Eater Meter Score of 184 because it saves over two miles of driving, almost a full square meter of land, and over 181 gallons of water, all without sacrificing a single bit of taste. (You can see the basic savings of air, land, and water for some of the most common foods in "Calculate Your Own Green Eater Meter Savings" on page 293 in the appendix, or see the full calculation sheet at https://omdfortheplanet.com/get-started/the-benefits.)

MY OMD STORY

Jenny Briesch

I started teaching kindergarten at MUSE the year they implemented the OMD program. At first, a lot of the parents thought we'd be starving their children. But over the past three years, the difference is just amazing—all the parents are on board now, because they see the benefits. Their kids eat vegetables now, whereas they didn't before. I can't tell you what a contrast that is with my previous school. There, the kids ate nothing but processed foods, so that's all they wanted. Here, I'm constantly amazed by how willing the kids are to try anything on their plate. They're also very energized by the water savings that we write on the board for every student. The kids that eat plant-based at home as well as at school have much higher totals every day. We talk about that: you could turn off the water while rinsing your toothbrush, delay flushing the toilet, take shorter showers—and it still wouldn't have the same impact as eating one plant-based meal a day.

Still, for me, OMD was a bit of a shock and a transition. When I came to MUSE, I was still eating meat—I was a total meathead. I was convinced that I had to have tons of protein to have energy. It took me about two years of doing OMD, slowly cutting down on meat, before I felt ready to ditch it for good. I just kept shrinking my portion sizes and looking for alternate meals whenever possible. Then I just went for it.

My friend from school, Melissa Pampanin, encouraged me to do a thirty-day challenge over the summer; I did it, and I never looked back. To get through the cravings, she made a suggestion that held me through the rough patches: Just eat veggies and fruit. In quantity. No limits. So if I ever really wanted to have a steak or a piece of chicken, I would head to the kitchen and eat a bunch of whatever veggie was on hand—and it worked! I'll never forget the image of Melissa tucking into a big bowl of watermelon—I learned I didn't have to be afraid of fruit, that fruit's sugar was bound up with fiber and was healthy, not bad for me.

Now, I still have cravings, and I can't seem to quit cheese. But I will get there! One day at a time. And it all started with OMD.

When you see those figures written down in black and white, you can imagine your environmental savings on a scale, as opposed to an all-or-nothing proposition. You can see your environmental savings growing and accumulating. Bit by bit, bite by bite, your choices are reclaiming the green heart of our planet.

If you'd like to keep a running total of your Green Eater Meter savings, you can print out a tally sheet from https://omdfortheplanet .com/get-started/the-benefits. On that page, you'll also find a way to calculate your savings over the longer term, forecasted out five, ten, fifty, and one hundred years (to slow climate change, protect glaciers, halt rising seas, promote ocean/forest/biodiversity regeneration, and more).

To get a quick sense of the relative differences in the environmental impact of different foods, check out "What Does It Take to Make . . ." on page 102 and the Greenhouse Gas Emissions chart below.

GREENHOUSE GAS EMISSIONS (per kilo of food, from low to high)[8]

Onion	0.17
Celery	0.18
Potatoes	0.18
Carrots	0.20
Zucchini	0.21
Cucumber	0.23
Beets	0.24
Pumpkins	0.25
Cantaloupe	0.25
Lemons and limes	0.26
Mushrooms	0.27
Apples	0.29
Pears	0.31
Green beans	0.31
Watermelons	0.32
Dates	0.32
Oranges	0.33
Kiwi fruit	0.36

Cauliflower	0.36
Grapes	0.37
Oats	0.38
Peas	0.38
Cherries	0.39
Almond/coconut milk	0.42
Peaches/nectarines	0.43
Figs	0.43
Apricots	0.43
Chestnuts	0.43
Tomatoes	0.45
Corn	0.47
Artichokes	0.48
Soybeans	0.49
Pineapples	0.50
Grapefruit/pomelo	0.51
Spinach	0.54
Garlic	0.57
Strawberries	0.58
Broccoli	0.60
Olives	0.63
Pinto beans	0.73
Soy milk	0.75
Chickpeas	0.77
Asparagus	0.83
Peanuts	0.83
Raspberries	0.84
Sesame seeds	0.88
Ginger	0.88
Cranberries/blueberries	0.92
Hazelnuts	0.97
Lentils	1.03

Herring	1.16
Milk (world average)	1.29
Avocados	1.30
Yogurt	1.31
Eggplant	1.35
Sunflower seeds	1.41
Cashew nuts	1.44
Walnuts	1.51
Pistachios	1.53
Almonds	1.54
Tuna	2.15
Rice	2.55
Eggs	3.46
Salmon	3.47
Cod	3.51
Chicken	3.65
Lettuce	3.70
Cream	5.64
Pork	5.77
Turkey	7.17
Shrimp	7.80
Cheese	8.55
Butter	9.25
Mussels	9.51
Swordfish	12.84
Lamb	25.58
Beef	26.61
Lobster	27.80
Buffalo	60

Invest! You Deserve High-Quality Ingredients

Investing in good pantry ingredients is always important when cooking, but it might be even more important when cooking vegan, since you're not using butter, cheese, or meat, which often have dominant flavors and textures. Investing in good-quality olive oil, vinegars, sea salt, and a good pepper grinder will make a big difference in taste.

Extra-virgin olive oil. This takes a little trial and error; when you taste one you like at a friend's home or a restaurant, jot down the name. And if you shop at a grocery store staffed by foodies, ask for recommendations. Olive oil should have its own distinct character—for example, fruity, a little peppery (that back-of-the-throat burn), or with a crushed-olive taste. Don't be afraid to sub in olive oil for milder-tasting oils in baking—for most baked goods, extra-virgin olive oil lends depth of flavor, but doesn't detract.

Vinegars. Every kitchen needs five vinegars to cover the whole spectrum of dishes: red wine vinegar, balsamic vinegar, apple cider vinegar, rice vinegar, and distilled white vinegar. With those five, you're golden. Artisanal balsamic vinegars are the best!

Sea salt. Sea salt doesn't just add flavor—because of its uneven, rough-hewn edges, it also adds texture. A pinch of sea salt takes any vegetable dish or salad up a notch.

Good pepper grinder. Nothing can compete with the flavor profile of freshly ground pepper. If you've never had one in your kitchen before, trust me—you will not go back to the simple shaker.

High-quality in-season vegetables. In plant-based cooking, vegetables are no longer the side dish bit players, they are now the stars on center stage—so opting for higher-quality, fresher ingredients is truly essential.

Getting All the Nutrition Bases Covered

As you're moving toward more of a whole-food, plant-based life-style, you might wonder about your nutrients—if you eat less meat, will you get everything you need? Well, we do know that a whole-food, plant-based diet comes with tons of health perks, starting with one that many of us struggle with: body weight. In a study of North American Seventh-day Adventists, a religious group that espouses vegetarianism, researchers found that the average plant-based eater's BMI was 23.6, compared to 28.8 for those who bucked their religious traditions and ate meat.[9] (For someone who is five feet nine, that's the difference between weighing 160 pounds and 195 pounds.) And we also know that those plant-based eaters have lower blood pressure and cholesterol, and less risk of developing type 2 diabetes and various types of cancer, not to mention serious digestive diseases.[10,11,12] So they must be doing something right!

Still, the emphasis here should be on the "whole food" part of the whole-food, plant-based diet—being a rice-pasta-bread vegan (or worse: a Diet Coke–and–french fries vegan) certainly won't give you any of those benefits. OMD is all about eating plenty of fruits and vegetables, nuts and seeds, some whole grains, and healthy fats. As you go, keep a close eye on the following nutrients—some plant-based eaters can fall short on these, but a few suggestions can help you make sure you don't. (Full disclosure: I take B_{12}, B complex, D_3, and magnesium, and I take an algae oil for omega-3, to make sure my bases are covered.)

B_{12}

RDA for adults: 2.4 mcg daily; during pregnancy: 2.6 mcg; during breastfeeding: 2.8 mcg[13]

Supplementing with this vitamin is a must, because B_{12} is found in foods of animal origin. The animals get it from bacteria that live in the soil, but because we overwash all our produce, we don't get as much, so plant-based eaters can pop up as deficient in B_{12} in research studies.[14]

While certain fermented foods such as tempeh and sauerkraut contain bacteria that produce B_{12}, there's not enough to cover the difference. You could get your RDA through B_{12}-fortified cereals and other foods, but if you're not consistently eating them, your B_{12} levels can fall. That's why health experts recommend a B_{12} supplement.[15] This becomes especially important after age fifty, when a dip in stomach acid and a substance called intrinsic factor can make it harder for everyone—not just those who are plant-based—to absorb B_{12}.

B_{12} is one of those vitamins you don't want to mess with. Among its many jobs, it helps produce DNA—in other words, the foundation of your cells, including your nerve cells and red blood cells. A deficiency can cause weakness, numbness in the feet and hands, depression, confusion, and even dementia. Catch it early enough, and supplements can reverse the symptoms, but a long-term deficiency can lead to irreversible damage, including brain damage—serious stuff.

Supplements tend to contain above-RDA levels, which is OK, because this vitamin is safe in higher amounts. Consult with your health-care provider about an appropriate dose.

Omega-3s

RDA of ALA (alpha-linolenic acid) for men: 1.6 g; for women: 1.1 g

Here's the deal with these fats: The type considered most effective at fighting inflammation, protecting your brain and heart, and staving off all types of chronic diseases are EPA and DHA, usually found in fish but also in vegan microalgae.[16] The type found in plants that you'd normally eat—walnuts, flaxseeds, hemp, and chia seeds—is ALA. Your body converts a little ALA to EPA and DHA, but sometimes not much, which is why plant-based eaters tend to have lower blood levels of EPA and DHA. Is this a problem? The research hasn't yet figured it out.

What we do know is that fish oil supplements are no sure bet, either—repeated meta-analyses of available data, involving hundreds of thousands of patients with heart disease, arthritis, and other chronic conditions, show conflicting results. Some studies showed benefit; some did not.[17] And if we keep in mind that fish oil supplements can be contaminated with heavy metals and persistent toxic pollutants such as PCBs, fish oil comes out as a net negative.

To be safe, the latest recommendation from the Academy of Nutrition and Dietetics is that plant-based eaters get a little more ALA than the suggested RDA—which is easy to achieve with an ALA supplement. You might consider a microalgae supplement providing 200 to 300 mg of DHA and EPA if you're pregnant, breastfeeding, or an older person with diabetes or another chronic disease, according to a 2013 research study in the *Medical Journal of Australia*.[18] (These groups have heightened omega-3 needs.)

PLANT-BASED SOURCES OF OMEGA-3S

One of the mistakes people can make when transitioning to a plant-based diet is eating too few healthy fats. Our bodies need enough fat to help form cell membranes and ensure good oxygen and blood flow through the body. Your daily omega-3 target should be at least 1.1 grams for women and 1.6 grams for men.

The essential fatty acid ALA is common in many plant-based foods; your body will use it to synthesize EPA and DHA, which are important for brain and heart health and for decreasing inflammation. Vegan DHA supplements, made from cultured microalgae, are also available online and in your local health foods store.

Canola oil
Chia seeds
Collard greens
Edamame
Flaxseed (oil or freshly ground seeds)*
Hempseed
Kidney beans
Miso *(ask at restaurants, because some misos are prepared with fish sauce)*
Mungo beans (aka urad dal or black lentil)
Pinto beans
Poppy seeds
Pumpkin seeds
Romaine lettuce
Sesame seeds (tahini)
Soy-based meat substitutes (ground "beef," "chicken" strips)
Soybeans (roasted)
Soy milk
Spinach
Tempeh
Tofu
Walnut (oil or nuts)*
Wheat germ oil
Winter squash

*best sources

Miso Is Amazing

M iso is amazing–this fermented soybean paste is a traditional ingredient in Japanese foods and boasts all kinds of beneficial vitamins, minerals, and isoflavones. Studies have proven that it can protect against colon, breast, liver, and gastric tumors and lower risk of stroke, and its dipicolinic acid can even protect against radiation injury. (A group of people living just a mile from where the atomic bomb was dropped in Nagasaki did not develop any acute radiation disease, and doctors later linked this to their miso consumption.) Miso's beneficial bacteria also help feed your gut lining and keep your microbiome stocked with friendly bugs. If you're not a fan of soy, you can also find chickpea miso.[19] I use chickpea miso as a base and toss in veggies and a few tablespoons of sun-dried tomato or sweet potato hummus for a quick soup. Yum!

Iodine

RDA: 150 mcg; during pregnancy: 220 mcg;
during breastfeeding: 290 mcg

If you regularly eat seaweed or use iodized salt, you're probably covered for this mineral. Iodine deficiency can cause thyroid issues, which can pose a problem for plant-based eaters. We tend to have a high intake of foods such as flaxseed, peanuts, pears, spinach, cruciferous vegetables, sweet potatoes, and strawberries, all of which are goitrogenic (meaning they can trigger thyroid goiters if you're not getting enough iodine). Supplementing with iodine should always be done under a doctor's supervision.

Calcium

RDA for women age 50 and younger (including those who are pregnant or breastfeeding) and men age 70 and younger: 1,000 mg; for women age 51 and older and men age 71 and older: 1,200 mg

Taking calcium supplements has become controversial, as several studies have linked them to dementia (in women)[20] and heart disease (in men)[21] who have some degree of preexisting cardiovascular disease. Some experts, such as Dr. Dean Ornish, allege that calcium supplements and animal products create acidic blood pH, which leaches calcium from the bones and leads to osteoporosis—meaning that dairy products do not make strong bones but actually make them weaker. Good plant-based sources of the mineral include tofu, calcium-enriched soy, almond and other nondairy milks, dried figs, sesame seeds and tahini, and tempeh. Calcium from some vegetables, such as kale, mustard and turnip greens, Chinese cabbage, and bok choy, is well absorbed. Calcium from other vegetables, such as spinach, beet greens, and Swiss chard, is not as well absorbed. Take care to ensure that you have enough vitamin D_3, as it also helps the body absorb calcium.

D_3

RDA for men and women up to age 70 (including women who are pregnant or breastfeeding): 15 mcg (600 IU); men and women age 71 and older: 20 mcg (800 IU)

Everyone—plant-based and animal-food eaters—has a hard time getting enough of this vitamin, which is produced when sunlight hits the skin. Plant-based sources are slim, so supplementation may be the best bet. You can get your D levels checked via a blood test; if you fall short, follow your health-care provider's advice about "restocking" your D stores. If your levels are good, look for D_3 supplements that provide 500 to 1,000 IU daily.

The Protein Question

Ah, the question every single plant-based eater gets, sometimes daily, or even multiple times a day. "How do you get enough protein?"

Oh, the anguish I've witnessed over this question. Here's the dirty secret about this obsession: we don't need a ton of protein, and we are eating waaaay too much right now. Men need about 56 grams of protein a day, and women need 46 grams. Right now, men are eating about twice what they need (100 grams), and women almost as much (70 grams). I'd say we have a lot of room to play around with that requirement.

Have you ever known anyone diagnosed as protein-deficient? And we are talking about a genuine medical diagnosis, rather than one by a well-meaning busybody. It's unlikely, because true protein deficiency (called kwashiorkor) almost never appears in developed nations. This is because protein deficiency really only happens when a person is starving to death and is deficient in virtually all nutrients.

Protein is necessary for a healthy body because it provides certain amino acids that our bodies do not naturally produce. These amino acids aid in everything from immune system response to nutrient transmission throughout the body to providing some of the building blocks for our skin, muscles, organs, even our hair and teeth. However, the amount of protein we require to function is much, much lower than is commonly thought.

So how did we become so obsessed with getting protein? I bet you can guess. That's right: the meat lobby. Like all savvy marketers, big animal agribusiness made sure that if they didn't have outright virtues to extol, they could make virtues out of what they did have. Meat offers a large amount of protein, so they decided that protein is the best—even the only—way to build muscle and become stronger. And anyone who doesn't consume enough protein (which is almost always conflated with meat, the same way "calcium" often translates to "milk") is probably anemic, weak, and frail. A meat-heavy diet is thus for "normal" people who want to be strong and healthy, and a vegan or vegetarian diet is for "weaklings."

The great big secret that meat marketers don't want you to know is that we can get everything we need (including protein and, yes, even calcium) from a diet entirely free of animal products. Protein can be found in all sorts of legumes and nuts, as well as in certain vegetables. Vegans and vegetarians are not wispy anemics; they can be just as strong and capable as any meat eater, and vegan athletes are now proving that performance levels are even higher on an all-plant diet. (As an executive producer of the film, I know I'm biased, but just watch *The Game Changers* if you want any proof—and motivation!)

Getting That Plant Protein

Protein is made of subunits called amino acids. A protein's quality, or "completeness," rests on its profile of "essential" amino acids—those are the ones our bodies can't make. Just like animal protein, soy products (such as tofu, tempeh, and edamame) and quinoa contain all the essential amino acids in decent amounts. (However, it takes a lot of quinoa to get the same amount of total protein as soy, because it's also so high in carbohydrates that the protein is somewhat diluted.) Other high-protein plant foods such as wheat, oats, and legumes are rich in some essential amino acids and low in others. Happily, by having a variety of plant proteins over the course of the day, you'll score all the essential amino acids in sufficient quantities. Make sure to have a few servings of at least one food from each group of essential amino acids so your body can adequately build protein.

rich in methionine/ low in lysine [22, 23]	rich in lysine/ low in methionine
Wheat	Black beans, chickpeas (garbanzo)
Rice	Oats
Hemp	Soy
Corn	Lentil
	Potato
	Peas

Remember: You don't have to have these "complementary protein foods" at the same meal, just throughout the course of the day. Here's how this translates to your plate:

- 🌏 Toss edamame, chickpeas, white beans, or any other beans (½ to 1 cup) into your salad.
- 🌏 Spread hummus (about ⅓ cup) over your sandwich.
- 🌏 Drink soy or pea protein milks (about 1 cup).
- 🌏 Make rice and bean pilafs.
- 🌏 Have black bean chili over rice.
- 🌏 Use tofu and tempeh.

The Scoop on Soy: Cooking with Tofu and Tempeh

Soy has a mixed reputation these days, but it's actually gotten kind of a bad rap. I used to be terrified of soy, but all the controversy about soy's estrogenic effects raising risks of breast or prostate cancer has been essentially debunked. "Organic soy products are safe and beneficial," says Dr. Dean Ornish. Organic soy products contain phytoestrogens, which resemble regular estrogen and bind to estrogen receptors but only weakly stimulate them. "It's somewhat like putting a key in a lock that doesn't open the lock but keeps the right key from opening it," says Dr. Ornish. "The net effect of soy is to reduce overall estrogen production." Since estrogen is linked to increased cell growth and proliferation—especially in breast cancer and prostate cancer—this phytoestrogenic effect tamps down that proliferation to help reduce the rate of these cancers. Dr. Ornish says while it's possible to eat so much soy that your estrogen production is increased, "this is generally more than most people would be consuming."

Research published in *JAMA* found that women who ate soy after their breast cancer were 32 percent less likely to have a recurrence and 28 percent less likely to die when compared with those who steered clear of soy.[24] Soy may also help reduce prostate cancer risk.[25] What's clear either way is that the least-processed soy products—tofu, tempeh, and soy milk—are likely much healthier than soy products that are heavily processed (such as tofu hot dogs, burgers, and isolated soy concentrates).

Soy can be one of the heartiest, most satisfying plant protein sources—but if you've never cooked with tofu or tempeh before, there can be a little learning curve. Here are a few pointers to keep it simple.

Tips for Tofu

Tofu is the blank canvas of plant proteins, extremely versatile and able to take on almost any flavor. You can try dry spice rubs (best for baking or roasting); marinating (depending on how porous the tofu is, more or less marinade will be infused); or simply letting the tofu absorb the flavors it's cooked in. Whether it's bananas and strawberries in a smoothie or spices in a curry, tofu is an excellent ingredient collaborator. Don't expect flavors to completely infuse throughout intact tofu—it's not that porous—but the smaller it's sliced or crumbled, the more flavor can be infused.

Tofu comes in various firmnesses. On the softer, moister end of the spectrum is "silken"; on the drier, firmer end is "extra-firm"; and there are levels in between. How do you decide what type to use? Think about the end result—the texture and moisture level of the dish you're making—and you'll have your answer.

Soft or Silken: Moistest, good for dips and smoothies, and can even be used as an egg replacement in recipes. (Check out Pagie Poo's Chocolate Mousse, page 278.)

For example: Add ⅓ to ½ cup silken tofu to your favorite smoothie recipes.

Medium-firm: Drain before using. Because it's still delicate and soft, it will break apart easily, so use this one in dishes that don't require stirring or rough handling.

For example: Drop it into miso soup.

Firm: Solid enough to stand up to gentle stir-frying (it'll still fall apart a little), and can be simmered into tomato sauces, curries, and other dishes. Firm tofu can also be crumbled and used somewhat like ricotta cheese in casseroles or as a substitute for scrambled eggs (check out Scrambled Tofu, page 205).

For example: For crumbles, remove the tofu from its container and use your hands to crumble it into pea-size pieces. Season it with olive oil, salt, and pepper and cook in a heavy-bottomed skillet over medium heat, stirring often, until browned. Or cook it with no-chicken broth. Use immediately, or keep refrigerated for a few days. Add to any recipe in place of ground meat or to your favorite stir-fry.

Extra-firm and Super-firm: The driest and most solid varieties, these types of tofu are also the most concentrated in protein. These are the ones to use in a vigorous stir-fry or for panfrying, and you can bake or roast them as well. (Check out Brad and Sandy's Sun-Dried Tomato and Asparagus Lasagna, page 250.)

For example: To roast, slice a block of extra-firm tofu into ¼-inch-thick slices, season with soy sauce or olive oil, salt, and pepper, and roast in a preheated 400°F oven until golden brown.

Tips for Tempeh

Tempeh is compressed and fermented whole soybeans, often mixed with barley or another whole grain. Tempeh is much firmer and nuttier than tofu. Because the soybeans are only partially cooked, you need to cook tempeh to make it more easily digested. Tempeh is delicious sliced, sprinkled with a little reduced-sodium soy sauce, and sautéed in olive oil. The strips can top a salad, go into a stew or curry, or be tossed with salt, pepper, and herbs and eaten as is—just the way you'd have a piece of chicken or fish.

As with tofu, tempeh can also be crumbled; just use your hand to crumble it into pea-size pieces. Season it with olive oil, salt, and pepper and cook in a heavy-bottomed skillet over medium heat, stirring often, until browned. Use immediately, or keep refrigerated for a few days. Add to any recipe in place of ground meat or to your favorite stir-fry.

Tempeh can also be marinated and baked. Slice or cube it, marinate at room temperature in your favorite marinade for 15 minutes to 2 hours, and bake in a preheated 375°F oven for about 20 minutes, until golden brown. Add to your favorite salad or serve as a side with any vegetables.

Ditch That Dairy: The Best Plant-Based "Milk"

It's a good time for vegan milks: well over half—58 percent—of all grocery store shoppers drink some kind of nondairy milk. After decades of just soy, rice, and almond milks, recently hemp, pea protein, and cashew milks are making a splash. (Pea protein milk is particularly tasty, with a nice, creamy mouthfeel.) They can all be used in smoothies, lattes and other hot drinks, cooking, and baking, and added to coffee and cereal.

Many parents are concerned about their kids missing out on cow's milk because it was such a solid source of protein. No problem. Just seek out higher-protein milks, of which there are plenty.

> *Almond milk.* A staple in almost every coffee shop, almond milk is truly mainstream now. Almond milk's nuttiness makes it a love-it-or-hate-it thing, but most find it an

enjoyable (and, helpfully, widely available) option. Almond also features in some "nut-blend" milks, which can disguise the nuttiness, if that's an issue.

Soy milk. Soy is one of the few plant proteins that is complete, so nutritionally, soy milk makes a good substitute for cow's milk. However, its slightly bean-y taste isn't for everyone. But whip it into a smoothie with fruit and other flavors, and the beaniness disappears—it makes for a richer-tasting drink than if you'd used cow's milk.

Pea protein milk. Made from yellow split peas, pea protein milk is also very rich and creamy—and its neutral taste makes it very versatile. Although it is high in protein, the protein is missing an essential amino acid, so it is not considered "complete." However, as we covered in "Getting That Plant Protein" (page 117), in combination with another plant protein, pea protein would get you pretty far toward meeting your protein needs.

Hemp milk. Compared to pea protein and soy milk, hemp milk has a slightly thinner consistency, with about half the protein (but more protein and essential fatty acids than other plant-based milks). Give it a try—its assertive flavor is something people tend to like or dislike.

Coconut milk. The creaminess of coconut milk makes it a good transitional milk for kids, and a great swap for half-and-half in your coffee. Canned coconut milk also lends a richness to dishes in which you might previously have used dairy cream, such as our Spinach–Sweet Potato Soup (page 215). (Note: Please read the cautions about coconut on page 123.)

Bottom line: You don't need dairy for strong bones—in fact, some preliminary research suggests that eating dairy for a lifetime may *weaken* your bones.[26] In a 2014 Swedish study of over sixty thousand women and forty-five thousand men published in the *British Medical Journal*, researchers found that drinking milk was not only linked to a higher risk of fractures (especially hip fractures), but that the more milk people drank, the higher their risk of mortality. In subsamples of another group, the researchers found that milk drinkers had higher levels of oxidative stress biomarkers in their urine and inflammation biomarkers in their blood.

But even if you've poured dairy milk on your cereal for years, all is not lost. "Eating a plant-based diet can help reverse the progression of osteoporosis in many people," says Dr. Dean Ornish, "especially when combined with aerobic exercise, resistance training, stress management techniques, low sodium (sodium promotes calcium loss in the urine), low caffeine (causes acidity, which also promotes calcium loss in urine and reduces calcium absorption), and sunshine/vitamin D_3." Ditch the dairy, and your bones will thank you.

Be Cautious With Coconut

As tempting as it may be to add some luscious coconut milk, oil, or cream to every dish, please think of coconut as an occasional treat, like birthday cake. Coconut oil is over 90 percent saturated fat! Even if you believe the as-yet-unproven theories about the supposed antimicrobial, immune-system-boosting wonders of coconut's medium chain fatty acids, take those MCFAs away, and that still leaves 45 percent straight saturated fat— weighing in at an impressive 2 percent more than lard itself. Tread cautiously!

SOME FAVORED PLANT-BASED MILK BRANDS

Milk is such a personal preference. What's too thin for some is refreshing for others; what's rich and creamy for some is gelatinous for others. The best thing to do when making the transition is just to jump in and experiment. Maybe join up with a few friends and do a side-by-side taste test, so you won't be on the hook for the whole cost. We had a blindfolded taste test with scores, which was a blast for the kids. Or try a new kind each week until you find "the one."

Here are some brands that are recommended often in online vegan communities. You might find some attractive alternatives here.

SOY-BASED
365 Unsweetened Organic Soy Milk (Whole Foods)
Alpro Organic Unsweetened Soy Milk
Eden Foods Unsweetened Soy Milk
Natur-a Unsweetened Organic Soy Milk
Simple Truth Unsweetened Soy Milk (Meijer/Kroger)
Vitasoy Protein Plus
WestSoy Organic Unsweetened Plain

OTHER
Aldi Unsweetened Vanilla Almond Milk
Blue Diamond Almond Breeze Almond Coconut Blend
Blue Diamond Almond Breeze Unsweetened Original
Califia Unsweetened Almond Milk
Kirkland Organic Unsweetened Vanilla Almond Milk
MALK Unsweetened Almond Milk

Silk Almond-Cashew Unsweetened Milk
Simple Truth Unsweetened Almond Milk (Meijer/Kroger)
Good Karma Unsweetened Flax Milk
Oatly! Oat Milk
Ripple Unsweetened Pea Milk

Make Your Own Nut Milk

What could be more empowering than creating your own milk, right there at home? Cashew milk is satisfying and creamy, and the homemade version boasts 6 grams of protein per cup, without all the yucky fillers or preservatives. Caveat: Don't try this with a standard blender—you need a high-powered one, like a Vitamix, or a food processor to get all the chunks out.

To Make Cashew-Hazelnut Milk: Put 1 cup raw cashews and ½ cup raw hazelnuts in a bowl, add water to cover, and set aside to soak for 8 hours. Drain and transfer to a blender with 4 cups filtered water, 5 pitted dates (and/or 1 teaspoon pure vanilla extract), and a pinch of salt. Blend until smooth, then strain through cheesecloth or a nut milk bag into a mason jar or other container with a tight seal. Store in the fridge for up to 2 days.

MASON JARS: THE WORLD'S BEST TO-GO CONTAINER

Mason jars are the perfect storage and to-go container. The best! You can get them in virtually any size–from a 2-ounce jar to ¼ pint (4 ounces) and all the way up to a gallon (128 ounces). You can't beat the price–you can find the pint jars for less than two bucks a piece. You can use them to can preserves, sauerkraut, even Mom Cameron's Chili Sauce (page 261). You can use them to transport chili to work. Just take off the top and pop the whole thing in the microwave. You can freeze soups or sauces in larger jars, and transport iced tea or coffee in smaller jars. There's even a stainless steel drinking lid made by EcoJarz that you can screw onto the top of the jar and sip from (find it at www.ecojarz. com). No more drinking out of stinky, chemical-leaching plastic cups for you–what could be better than drinking clean filtered water out of glass?

I also sometimes keep those tiny jars from the honey or jam you get at restaurants or hotels–they're perfect for salad dressing or hummus. My favorite thing to do when I travel is to take a salad in a widemouthed mason jar and several of these little tiny 1-ounce jars (TSA-ready size) filled with my dips. Then I enjoy them during the flight (and try to remember to rinse them out before I go through customs!).

Stocking Your OMD Pantry

Our weekly, biweekly, and monthly shopping lists depend on the season, the kids' activities, what projects Jim and I are working on, and many other factors. But I have found that having certain staples in the house ensures that we can always whip up a plant-based meal on the fly. We have a big storage freezer, so we try to stock up on certain favored items; if you can get one, it can yield big food savings in the long run. Also, buying in bulk and cases will usually yield 10 to 20 percent off in some co-ops, on Thrivemarket .com, and even on Amazon.

We order bread and bagels online from Sami's Bakery in Florida and store them in the freezer. This allows us to purchase once every month and a half to two months or longer. Fresh produce and other perishable items (fruits, veggies, fresh almond milk, yogurt, cheeses, dips, etc.) are purchased weekly or biweekly. Pantry items like beans, sauces, oils, teas, etc., are purchased as and when needed, with certain staples available in quantity at all times. For example:

- 🌍 Kidney beans—at least 6 cans or more in the pantry
- 🌍 Box of soups (tomato or vegetarian no-chicken broth)—at least 4 boxes of each
- 🌍 Olive oils and vinegars—at least 2 bottles or more
- 🌍 Shelf-stable plant-based milk—2 backup packs of almond, coconut, soy, pea protein, and nut blends

(See the OMD Master Pantry List on page 295.)

Buy It Fresh (When You Can)

As I said, there's nothing wrong with frozen—or even canned— veggies if it makes OMD easier for you. Especially when it comes to beans, some people swear by the ease of cans. But in general, the fresher the fruit or vegetable, the more nutrients it contains. The tastiest and most nutritious fruit and vegetables are:

- 🌏 in season in your area
- 🌏 picked at peak ripeness, or at a mature enough stage that they ripen to perfection on your kitchen counter

While picking it yourself is the only surefire way to know how fresh your produce is, produce from strictly local farmers' markets or CSAs may be incredibly fresh as well. (Just ask the farmer when it was harvested.)

But most of us get our produce at grocery stores, which means you'll have to do some sleuthing to get the freshest picks.

- 🌏 *Look for local.* Even mainstream supermarkets may carry a few local fruits or vegetables—check for signs and ask. But just because it's local doesn't guarantee freshness; look them over carefully. (The "Buying and Storing Guide for Select Fruits and Vegetables" on page 131 tells you what to look for.)
- 🌏 *Stick to seasonal and semi-local.* Even if the food isn't local, if it's seasonal and comes from a state in your general region of the country, it might not have traveled for too many days. Sure, you might get a yen for peaches in January and pay top dollar for those flown from South America, but you're taking your chances on freshness (and kind of defeating the purpose, climate-wise).
- 🌏 *Use your eyes, nose, and hands—and know your produce.* A soft, wrinkled mango? It's probably at perfect ripeness. A soft, wrinkled apple? Probably past its prime. (Cut it up and put it in the freezer to chuck in a smoothie later.) Recognize high-quality fruits and vegetables, and you'll come home from

the market with great stuff. Our "Buying and Storing Guide for Select Fruits and Vegetables" (page 131) fills you in on the more popular fruits and vegetables. Most produce should have a little give to the touch—only apples should be seriously hard. Punctures are a no-no, but blemishes may or may not be a problem. For example, small blemishes on oranges aren't an issue, but soft spots are.

Again—think frozen. In studies comparing fresh and frozen fruits and vegetables picked up at supermarkets, there's generally no difference in vitamin and mineral content. That's because most frozen vegetables are frozen immediately after they're picked, helping them retain their nutrients.[27,28]

Make It Last

You can get away with shopping just once a week and still have nutritious and tasty produce by following these tips:

- Buy both ripe and unripe fruit (including tomatoes). That way, you can enjoy the ripe fruit the first few days after your shopping trip, while allowing the other fruit to ripen on your counter.
- Some types of fruit are always sold ripe, such as apples, berries of all types, citrus, grapes, and watermelon. If you're going to eat them within twenty-four hours, it's fine to leave them on the counter, but otherwise, refrigerate them.
- You can purchase the following fruits at various stages of ripeness: bananas, cantaloupe, honeydew, kiwi, mango, papaya, pears, and tomatoes. Ripen them on your counter, uncovered; to speed things up, place them in a paper bag. (But don't use plastic—it will make them rot.) Once ripe, either eat them right away or refrigerate them in a glass container. The exception: tomatoes, which lose flavor if refrigerated.[29]

🌍 Stock up on long-lasting fruits and vegetables: apples, carrots, celery, citrus, onions, and radishes. Keep this produce wrapped and refrigerated, and it should still be fine more than a week (possibly weeks) later. Potatoes also have longevity if kept in a cool, dark spot—but don't refrigerate them, because their starches will start converting to sugars.

Refuse the Big 5

Little things add up. We think, *It won't matter that much if I use this one bag/one straw/one coffee cup/one plastic bottle.* What we really have to think about is what happens when one hundred, one hundred thousand, or one hundred million people in the world think the same thing. Consider:

- 380 billion plastic bags, sacks, and wraps are used in the United States each year.
- 3 million plastic bottles are used every *hour* in the United States. Less than 30 percent are recycled.
- 500 *million* straws are used every day in the United States.
- 25 billion Styrofoam cups are used each year in the United States.
- By 2050, plastic in the oceans will outweigh fish.

It all adds up, and every little bit we can do and demonstrate to others will help.

What are some things that we can all do? We can start by politely refusing the Big 5:

1. Plastic shopping bags
2. Plastic water bottles
3. To-go cups
4. To-go containers
5. Straws and utensils

Buying and Storing Guide for Select Fruits and Vegetables

This list will get you started with some of the more commonly eaten produce. Good sources of similar information are the extension service websites of Penn State, the University of Maine, and many other universities.

General tips for storing fruits and vegetables in the refrigerator[30]:

- Make sure they are dry before storing; otherwise, the moisture will cause them to rot. Wash just before eating or cooking with them.

- Store them whole; cut or slice just before cooking or serving. Otherwise, they lose nutrients and deteriorate more quickly.

- Store them in their original packaging—for example, keep spinach in its bag or clamshell (hard plastic container), berries in their clamshell, etc. These packages are designed to help produce last. (Note: while this can extend the shelf life of produce, I still prefer to use glass containers whenever possible, then recycle the original packaging.)

- If you don't have the original packaging (i.e., you bought the produce at a farmers' market), follow the directions on the chart on the next page. Use glass containers.

If you eat fruit or vegetables cold, right out of the fridge, you'll miss out on some of the flavor. Bring to room temperature by removing them from the fridge an hour before eating.

In general, we try to steer clear of plastic whenever possible, both to avoid the xenoestrogens they contain and the excess waste they create. To cut down on waste, we buy spinach in the big clamshells—and we constantly reuse them. If we go to a store that has spinach in bulk, we take a mesh bag to bring it home. We then wash and dry the spinach and store it in a glass container.

Another idea from a bygone era that needs to be brought back: 100 percent cotton flour sacks. In the days before salad spinners, Mom washed her lettuce and let it dry on a towel, then lightly wrapped it in flour sacks and put the whole thing in the crisper. In our house, I wash the lettuce, spin it, and put it in glass containers to store in the fridge, where it stays fresh for a week or longer.

FRUIT	
Apples[31]	Should be ... Very hard, taut, unwrinkled skin, with no soft or dark spots Store ... In a glass bowl, in the crisper (aka hydrator) in your refrigerator For best quality, eat within ... 2 weeks
Blueberries[32]	Should be ... Firm, dark blue/deep purple with a silvery finish called the "bloom" (its natural protective coating) Store ... In their own package, or a glass container For best quality, eat within ... 5 days
Cantaloupe	Should be ... A little soft on the stem end, which should also have a scent Store ... On the counter, if the melon needs to ripen (if it has just a faint scent and barely yields to the touch at the stem end). Refrigerate ripe melon, covered or uncovered, or cut up the fruit and store in an airtight container; store in the crisper/hydrator. For best quality, eat within ... 5 days
Grapes	Should be ... Firm but not hard, unwrinkled, ideally with a powdery-white "bloom" (its natural protective coating) Store ... In a glass bowl lined with a paper towel to absorb moisture For best quality, eat within ... 1 week
Oranges and Grapefruit[33,34,35]	Should be ... Heavy for its size, unwrinkled at the top (or elsewhere). Oranges may "regreen"–develop green areas due to a reaction to warm weather when on the vine–that's

fine; it doesn't mean they aren't ripe. Grapefruit should be slightly oval-shaped with a somewhat flat top and glossy skin–the thinner, the better.

Store . . . In the refrigerator's crisper/hydrator in their mesh bag or an open flour sack (don't seal it or they'll rot)

For best quality, eat within . . . 3 weeks

Peaches[36]

Should be . . . Slightly soft, especially at the "seam," heavy, with a slight perfume (if ripe). Yellow peaches should be yellow, white peaches white–both can have a red blush. Avoid those with a green tinge–they are too immature and may not ripen.

Store . . . On the counter, if they need to ripen–leave uncovered or place in a paper (never plastic) bag. Refrigerate ripe peaches in the crisper/hydrator in a glass bowl or flour sack

For best quality, eat within . . . 2 days

Strawberries[37] **Should be** . . . Firm, bright red with no–or just a faint touch of–white or green (otherwise, they won't be sweet). Stems should be fairly moist.

Store . . . On the counter in a cool spot, if you'll eat them within 24 hours. At about 60°F, levels of the antioxidants vitamin C and anthocyanins (which give the berries their red hue) increase, according to a University of São Paulo study. Otherwise, refrigerate in the crisper/hydrator in a glass container; if sold in a paper container, remove and place in bowl lined with paper towels to absorb moisture. You can loosely cover with a paper towel–but it should not be airtight.

For best quality, eat within . . . 2 to 3 days

VEGETABLES

Asparagus

Should be . . . Firm, with medium to thick stalks that are nearly completely green; tips should be closed and not wilted.

Store . . . Cut about ¼ inch off the stem end. Wash in lukewarm water a few times. Dry carefully. Stand the stalks in a jar or thick-bottomed glass filled with 2 inches of cold water, loosely cover the tops with a paper towel, and place in the crisper/hydrator of your fridge. Otherwise, just wrap the stem ends in a moist paper towel, place in a glass container, and refrigerate in the crisper/hydrator.

For best quality, eat within . . . 1 to 2 days

Beets, Carrots, and Radishes [38]	**Should be** . . . Firm, somewhat even and smooth. If the greens are attached, they should look fresh, not wilted. **Store** . . . In the crisper/hydrator of the fridge in a flour sack. Remove the greens before storing. Keep beet greens in a separate sack. **For best quality, eat within** . . . 2 weeks, possibly longer
Broccoli [39]	**Should be** . . . Dark green, even with a bluish tone with firm, tight buds. Avoid yellow buds–they mean the broccoli is past its prime. **Store** . . . In a flour sack in the crisper/hydrator in the fridge. We also cut broccoli and cauliflower and store in glass containers for convenience of grabbing quickly and adding to dishes. **For best quality, eat within** . . . About 4 days
Cauliflower [40]	**Should be** . . . Heavy for its size, white or off-white (or, for pigmented varieties, bright light green or purple), without blemishes or spaces between the curds. Leaves should be fresh and taut. **Store** . . . In a flour sack in the crisper/hydrator in the fridge. **For best quality, eat within** . . . About 4 days
Kale [41,42]	**Should be** . . . Moist, firm, richly colored green leaves–no yellowing or browning. Whether curly, dinosaur (pebbly), or other varieties, the small to medium leaves are the most tender. **Store** . . . In a flour sack in the crisper/hydrator in the fridge. **For best quality, eat within** . . . 5 days
Mushrooms	**Should be** . . . Small to medium for their particular variety (i.e., small portobellos will be a lot bigger than small button mushrooms). Caps should be fairly uniform in color, and either completely sealed around the stem or just slightly open. **Store** . . . In a paper bag in the crisper/hydrator in the fridge. **For best quality, eat within** . . . 5 days
Salad greens (lettuce, spinach)	**Should be** . . . Firm, taut, moist leaves, without yellowing or sliminess. **Store** . . . Iceberg: Wrapped in a flour sack bag in the crisper/hydrator in the fridge. Spinach and other greens: Clean and

dry; store in a glass container or loosely wrapped in a flour sack in the crisper/hydrator in the fridge.

For best quality, eat within . . . Head of iceberg: Up to 2 weeks. Head of romaine: 10 days. Spinach: 3 to 5 days. Other salad greens: 1 to 3 days.

Tomatoes	**Should be . . .** Ripe: Firm but not rock hard, with a deep color (i.e., red tomatoes should be deeply red; yellow tomatoes an orangey-yellow–however, some paler yellow tomatoes will stay that color, and some green varieties are ripe when green). Not quite ripe: Very firm, with a green tinge that usually disappears as it ripens. Avoid soft tomatoes and/or those with blemishes and punctures. **Store . . .** On the counter–don't refrigerate them, or they will lose flavor. **For best quality, eat within . . .** Ripe: Eat immediately. Otherwise, 1 or more days, depending on when they ripen.

Just Start Stacking Those Sandbags

Dr. David Katz uses a great image to describe the fight against climate change: picture the whole community pulling together to build a levee before a storm. "Nobody builds the whole levee alone . . . but if you're stacking a sandbag, you're part of the solution," he says. "And if enough of us stack bags of sand, before you know it, we've got a levee, and factors conspiring against the fate of the planet begin to recede.

"But that's really *all* you need to do—stack a sandbag," he says. Here are some "sandbags" Dr. Katz suggests, all of which we can easily do with OMD:

 Eat more plants and less animal food.

 Teach your children the reasons why this is important.

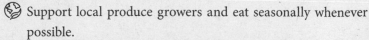 Support local produce growers and eat seasonally whenever possible.

🌏 Spread that message to schools (for example, by being on a wellness committee; go to the OMD website https://omdforthe planet.com/take-action/3-ways-to-help for our healthy school lunch toolkit).

🌏 Talk about it with your friends and on social media.

🌏 Encourage your favorite restaurants to add more plant-based menu items—and find out how to graciously do this with the restaurant toolkit on the OMD website https://omdforthe planet.com/take-action/3-ways-to-help.

🌏 Contribute to an environmental organization that recognizes the link with plant-based eating.

🌏 Create a good vegetarian recipe (or many) and share it online.

"The job seems overwhelming when you think you've got to do it alone," says Dr. Katz. "But we're not alone. That is both our greatest challenge and our greatest opportunity." By keeping OMD in the forefront of your mind, you can start influencing the people all around you, and together we can all become more in tune with the ways our diet can play a huge role in safeguarding our beautiful planet.

Now that you have all the info you need to start implementing OMD, it's time to go for it. Let's start!

chapter 5

One Meal a Day

You're off on your OMD journey! And as you get more comfortable with plant-based cooking, you can start to build in plant-based snacks or desserts, experiment with plant-based baking, or even try out a fully plant-based weekend every once in a while.

In a 2017 analysis published in the journal *Climatic Change*, researchers from three universities determined that making just one swap—swapping beef for kidney beans—could help us achieve up to *75 percent* of our Paris Agreement goals.[1]

That's before we adopt any other changes, even in our use of fossil fuels. Before we change fuel standards, increase solar or wind power, or cut down on overpopulation.

Three-quarters of the way there. Just with that one change!

We *can* make a difference. OMD can be your family's very concrete, very quantifiable way of saving the world.

Let's talk about all the ways that you can incorporate OMD into your life.

The Beauty of the Gentle Start

Kathy Freston, bestselling author of *The Lean*, is a good friend and part of the OMD brain trust, and she came to speak with the MUSE community when we were transitioning to plant-based lunches. I was sitting in the audience listening to her story, just blown away. Kathy is a gorgeous woman, a former model turned author, who has written several books about plant-based eating. Her own journey began when she saw a pamphlet about the torture endured by cows during slaughter, and then her very vital father's death at sixty-four. He'd been a big fan of meat, which she was soon to realize was extremely carcinogenic, and the one-two punch hit her very hard. She had an epiphany: *I don't want to eat that anymore.* She decided in a moment, but it took her three years to go completely plant-based. "It was really hard," she said to our community, and the honesty was refreshing. While some people flip a switch and go all in, many more people struggle a bit with the transition and have to work at it—like Kathy.

To see Kathy now, you'd think she's been plant-based from birth. Talk about glow—the woman is *illuminated* from within. During her modeling years, she'd always struggled with her weight, but since going plant-based, those struggles are now over. Someone in the audience at MUSE asked her how she started. "I just started with just the one meal on Saturdays. And then I did another one on Tuesdays. And then over time, I leaned into it," she said. "You don't have to do it overnight. Some people do. But it's hard.

"You have cravings for things, and then you're out with people, and they look at you weird," she recalled. "You have to find some friends to do it with you and get a support system. And you just lean a little bit further. You just try this, and then the next week you try that."

Up until that point, I'd been convinced that people should become plant-based all in one big jump—no time to lose for your health and the earth. Yet I could see that that approach was causing major pushback in my life, generating major resistance from my kids and my siblings. And here Kathy was, having taken three years to make the same transition, being open and honest about how hard it was—and people were hanging on her every word. And now she's a spokesperson for it. Her empathy and understanding were palpable and inspiring.

Kathy's story was a great reminder for me that we all learn and change in different ways, and perfection is the enemy of progress. Everyone can tailor OMD to their own lives—the emphasis is on *what works*. What works best for you, your cravings, your family, your work schedule—everything. Here are a few options you might consider—pick one of these, or create your own OMD approach. No wrong answers. (If you'd like to follow a more prescribed approach to OMD, check out the 14-Day OMD Transition Plan, page 164.)

Find a Buddy

This is super important. When Jim and I started this journey, we had each other—and that really helped. Having someone to help you find plant-based foods locally, brainstorm solutions, stay motivated—even share recipes and coupons—can be a tremendous help when you're first making the shift. Ideally, this will be a partner or someone in your house, or a dear friend. But even if you can't find anyone physically close, you can always find like-minded souls online. (Go to https://www.facebook.com/OMD4thePlanet/ to get support from my team and me and to connect with other people, families, and even schools that are doing OMD, just like you.)

Use the Five-Second Rule

The summer I was working on the book, I ran across Mel Robbins's TED Talk, "How to Stop Screwing Yourself Over." A great title, and so applicable to what we do when we're trying to make major change. Her five-second rule is such a great way to keep yourself on track, break unconscious habits, and stop reaching for the cheese. What is it, in a nutshell? "If you have an impulse to act on a goal, you must physically move within five seconds, or your brain will kill the idea."

You might just put the cheese down and shut the fridge door. You might walk directly to the fruit dish. You might make yourself reach for the hummus instead—whatever positive action you can take in five seconds. Try it. I have found it to be really effective at keeping me focused on my goals. (Check Mel out at http://melrobbins .com/the-5-second-rule/. Her book *The 5 Second Rule* is great.)

Steer Clear of Your Darlings

In the beginning, when we first went plant-based, we thought, "We'll just order a vegan pizza." And it was not good. In fact, I think the word the kids used was "disgusting." But things have changed so much in five years—including their palates. If you are a pizza lover, don't go from extra-cheesy sausage pizza to one topped with veggies and Daiya vegan cheese shreds in one leap—you might get turned off.

I'm not going to lie: cheese is tough. It's a very hard texture and taste to duplicate in plant food. However, there have been *enormous* strides in the past few years, and there are some absolutely amazing plant-based cheeses out there today. As your palate adjusts, I heartily recommend Kite Hill, Follow Your Heart, and Miyoko's Creamery cheeses, which you can get at most Whole Foods and Wegmans supermarkets; even Walmart and local grocery stores are starting to carry many plant-based options. Miyoko's has about fifteen flavors, with special offerings during the holidays, and they will ship directly to you. You can stir Miyoko's directly into hot pasta shells, and voilà—you have mac and cheese. Some are great for melting into a grilled cheese, some are great for just eating. (Check out a list of more of our favorite brands on page 295.)

Before you dive straight into any plant-based cheese, though, I encourage you to work with a recipe or two from chapter 7. Often the way they're prepared and the foods that surround them have a big impact on how they end up tasting.

Or Go Ahead and Pick a Stand-In

Some people have zero trouble with transition, especially with some of the more processed vegan "meats," like "chicken" fingers or faux lunch meats—the consistency of the originals are so synthetic to start that the substitutes don't feel like a hard stretch.

Takeout Is Your Friend

While you're in your OMD transition, indulge yourself in a little takeout. Stick with ethnic restaurants—Indian, Japanese, Chinese, Mexican, Italian, and Greek all have wonderful plant-based options. Chipotle is a no-brainer, plenty of vegan options there, especially with their delicious sofritas (GMO-free tofu, braised in a spicy broth with chipotle chiles, roasted poblano peppers, and a mix of Mexican spices). Other fast food options: oatmeal with blueberries and nuts at Starbucks, black bean soup at Panera, veggie subs and minestrone soup at Subway. You can even eat any bean-based dish at Taco Bell by ordering it "fresca"—they remove the sour cream and cheese and replace it with pico de gallo.

Toss That Ground Beef

One time I walked into the house and got a big whiff of grilled meat. *Oh, crud, they're making hamburgers*, I thought. Turns out, it was a Beyond Burger brand plant-based burger, which was meticulously designed to look, taste, and smell exactly like beef—and boy, does it!

Another time, on Easter Sunday, I walked into the house and smelled burgers again. I had a big Easter basket in my hands and Jim said, "Put that down, babe, you have to taste this." I'm thinking, *What are you doing?? Why are you doing this??* I see this big mound of "bleeding" ground beef sitting on the counter, and a bunch of sliders stacked up on a platter. I was dumbfounded.

Turns out, they were Impossible Burgers—we'd gotten some "raw" meat from Tal Ronnen, the amazing vegan chef at Crossroads

Kitchen in Los Angeles, to make at home. I thought for sure they were real burgers. I actually can't even eat them because they taste too much like real meat, but the rest of the family loves them.

Ground beef is one of the easiest meats to fake, which is great news because it is one of the biggest offenders in overall environmental damage, from greenhouse gas emissions to land use to water consumption. Doctoring veggie "beef" crumble into chili, lasagna, and tacos is so easy. Every once in a while, our friends Sandy and Brad, the plant-based caterers on the *Avatar* set, will throw some Beyond Beef into their lasagna (see page 250). It's a hearty way for people to transition away from beef.

If your family has sensitive palates, and you think they'll pick up on the swap, start by swapping out one-quarter of the meat in a recipe for the plant-based alternative, then half, then three-quarters—then go completely plant-based and see if they pick up on it. If they're not super fussy, just go all in on individual recipes where the swaps are easy. They'll likely never notice.

Try a Protein Progression

If you have a reluctant OMD-er in the house and they're not budging, you could try an even smaller baby step to a protein with a smaller footprint than beef. (Again, not very hard to do.) Any click toward the lower end of impact is a step in the right direction. (Moving from beef to chicken cuts 80 percent of the land use and 90 percent of the greenhouse gas emissions.)

For example, your protein progression could be something like this:

Beef → pork → chicken → egg → salmon → tofu → beans
Beef broth → chicken broth → veggie broth or faux chicken
broth (such as vegetarian no-chicken broth from Imagine
Foods)

Bacon → turkey bacon → faux bacon

Beef hot dogs → turkey hot dogs → vegan Alpha Dog

Don't get caught in the trap of thinking that free-range, grass-fed, organic beef is better than industrial meat. In fact, it's much worse for the environment. Methane from the fermentation in grass-fed cows' stomachs is one-third more pronounced than in grain-fed cattle. Also, remember those Rigiscan tests the college athletes took? (Turn back to page 39 if you want a refresher.) Their meat- and dairy-based meals had been made with the highest-quality animal products available, and those primo cuts of meat still made a huge difference in their penile circulation *after just one meal*!

Then try to think about ways to *add* vegetables and fruits to a meal. If someone in your family is insisting on a veggie omelet, add extra broccoli, spinach, mushrooms, onions, tomatoes. Cut down the animal-to-vegetable ratio—then start making it with one less egg every time.

Triple Up Those Lunches

Double or even triple the amount of fruit and/or vegetables you send to school in your kid's lunches each day, even if they come home uneaten at first. Slowly change the standard of what your kids see as their "normal" lunch. Cut vegetables into chunks and make veggie skewers; send them in with plant-based ranch, Caesar, soy sauce, or liquid aminos (an unprocessed version of soy sauce that's just soybeans and water; Bragg is a really good brand). Indulge in berries for a fruit salad. Create a yogurt dip, or even send a small amount of raspberry syrup or a tiny drop of maple syrup for dipping. Send along a set of chopsticks (also good for little ones' tactile and sensory input!).

OUR OMD STORY

Chrissy and Stuart Bullard

We have five people in our family, and five different ways of eating. Honestly, different bodies want different foods! Our two youngest sons have never really been into meat, so doing OMD is no problem for them. When the OMD program first came to MUSE, my older one was in first grade, and he had eaten meat his whole life (and he still eats a bit). At the beginning, I got some of the recipes from school so he could get used to the food. The seed-to-table program at school really helped him understand where food comes from and how it's made. He's only in fourth grade now, but at a young age he became really aware of what he was putting into his body and what it was doing to his body. I think it's making him aware of all health issues: he's asking questions like, "Why would people smoke a cigarette?"

In the beginning, I wondered why the school was doing this—but when I learned the rationale, I understood. Then I watched what it did to the kids. The more our kids were introduced to it, the more we wanted to be healthy too. Stuart was raised in Pittsburgh; his father owned a barbecue restaurant. When you're raised eating certain foods, you normally just carry on and teach your kids to eat those foods too. The OMD program brought new things into our household. Our son would come home and say, "I want to make kale chips!" We wanted to support him, so we went out to get the supplies and he would teach us how to make things. One day, he said, "I want radishes—I love radishes." We were like, "What kid likes radishes??" But OMD does that—it opens your kid up to foods you may not think they would like. Thing is, how would we know? When your child is exposed to more food (especially if they can grow those foods), it really broadens their horizons. All of our health has improved–Stuart has lost weight and feels stronger and has more energy; now when he eats meat, he can really tell how it just drags him down. He probably felt like that for years but just didn't realize it was the meat. Chrissy feels sharper and doesn't *need* to drink coffee anymore (she still likes to!). The best part is how the kids are leading the way–they're showing us how good plant-based eating truly is.

Reunite with PB&J

Fall back in love with peanut butter and jelly, but dress it up to make it feel more adult. No need to stick with PB—look at all the diverse nut butter options out there: almond, cashew, NuttZo blend. Same for the jams—get creative. Think preserves, compote, even cranberry sauce! Mix in hemp hearts with the peanut butter. Make peanut butter squares on crackers, and top with a berry or two. Mix the peanut butter with honey and layer it on apple circles, or just spread on some cashew or almond butter. I sometimes make open-faced apple sandwiches, layering apple, nut butter, berries, and bananas on top. (Check out Mom Cameron's Chili Sauce on page 261 for an interesting twist.)

Experiment With Nut Butters

Once you've tried some of the nut butter sandwich options, branch out. Almond, cashew, and peanut butter, as well as tahini (made from ground sesame seeds), are so versatile.

> 🌿 *Smoothie bolster.* Add a tablespoon or two to a smoothie—the extra calories, healthy fat, and other nutrients round out a breakfast smoothie, turning it into an energizing meal.

🌎 *Quick snack.* Pair with fruit (banana, apple, pear, dried apricot), a raw vegetable (celery, carrots), or crackers for an easy snack.

🌎 *Dip or dressing.* Here's our basic dressing formula: Mix three parts nut butter, two parts apple cider vinegar, and one part water and season with salt and pepper. And here's a dressing that makes any cooked vegetable or salad rich and creamy: Combine two parts tahini with one part rice vinegar or fresh lemon juice and add water a bit at a time until the dressing reaches desired consistency (it is impossible to say how much water exactly, since thickness of tahini varies so much). Season with salt and pepper and, if you like, add a little crushed garlic. Great on roasted cauliflower, any salad greens, or coleslaw.

Make Friends with Your Knife

Plant-based eating *can* go wrong if you eat too much processed food (vegan hot dogs, potato chips, and the like). However, if vegetables are always prominent in your meal—either taking center stage or mixed into dishes—you are on the right track. A common complaint about eating plant-based is that it takes more time than throwing a piece of meat on the grill. One of the best ways to cut back on vegetable prep time is by using a sharp, well-balanced knife.

Chef's knife: 8 inches long; handles slicing, dicing, mincing, and chopping.

Utility knife: 4 to 6 inches long; easier to handle for smaller fruits and vegetables.

Paring knife: used for peeling and coring.

Ideally, shop for these in person, picking up the knives to gauge how comfortable they are. You're going to be doing more chopping overall, so invest in a butcher block cutting board (no worries about cross-contamination when you're plant-based) or just get a bunch of cheap cutting boards at IKEA to keep things simple.

Treat Meat Like Cigarettes

Think of cutting down on meat the way some people think of cutting down on smoking: Start by cutting out the one meal where you don't even really "need" that meat. Maybe it's the slice of salami at the office party, or the extra slice of cheese on your sandwich at lunch. Then think about swapping out options from the menu—maybe cut the cheeseburger first (of course!), but rather than go straight to the vegan option, maybe you move first to the chicken breast or turkey burger, *then* to the veggie burger. And always remember that any animal product will not help your health in any way.

Find a Few Faves and Stick with Them

Keep it easy on yourself when you start. If you find a few recipes that you love right away, terrific. Get them into your normal rotation, and stay on the lookout to add more. We all gravitate toward things we know we like. Work up to adding new meals as you get more confident about OMD.

CHILI AS THE ULTIMATE GATEWAY DISH

The chili on page 230 is such a crowd-pleaser, it won't even register as OMD. I've been making it for as long as I've been with Jim. My kids are always asking, "Mom, when are you going to make your chili again?" And the crazy thing is, I don't even eat it, because I have an issue with onions, and I have to put six onions in there, chopped up. I wear sunglasses and gloves when I chop them and would wear a HAZMAT suit if I had one. So it is definitely a labor of love.

Jim's mother was the one who created the original recipe. She was in Canada, there was a blizzard outside, and she didn't have tomato paste—but she did have a can of Campbell's tomato soup. She used that, with some ground beef and onions and kidney beans, and the family said, "This is the best chili you've ever made." So she continued to make it that way.

When Jim and I got together, he said, "Babe, you've got to get my mom's chili recipe." Happily! I got it, I made it, and then I shaved out the Campbell's and started using organic tomato soup. Then we phased out ground beef and started putting in ground turkey. And when we went plant-based, there was a moment of, *What now? How can we mess with our beloved chili?*

I experimented with quinoa, which was really good. Then we tried rice. And then we found Beyond Meat "beefy" crumbles, and now you honestly just can't tell the difference. Non-plant-based people eat it and they have *no idea*. I've made it so many times now; very often I will make two batches of it because it's just gone within two days. Jim loves the leftovers, and the kids even eat it for breakfast. That's an OMD everyone can get behind.

Use Your Slow Cooker

Slow cookers have revolutionized weeknight cooking. You can almost be the worst chef in the world, and your slow cooker will hide a multitude of sins.

To get started, you need a slow cooker, of course. While any slow cooker will work, the Instant Pot is all the rage and is definitely one of the most versatile and powerful of the bunch because it works as a slow cooker and can also pressure cook, sauté, and perform other cooking functions. (See "Five Brilliant Instant Pot Hacks" on page 233 to learn how to use yours to make plant-based staples like applesauce, beans, rice, yogurt, and stewed tomatoes.)

If you have enough space in your freezer, you can prep a couple of weeks' worth of meals at once. Rather than use zip-top bags, which could leach plastic into your food, invest in a bunch of glass containers (we use Anchor Hocking Bake 'N Take containers) or an easily stackable size and shape of mason jar. Enlist the help of cooking compadres—kids, partner, roommates—set aside a weekend afternoon, create an assembly line, then get chopping. (Be sure to label the containers with their contents and the date so you can keep your inventory fresh.)

Take OMD to School

At the start of every school year—or shoot, all year long—make an issue out of it . . . be that squeaky wheel. Ask, "What kind of vegetarian options do you have for kids?" Often kids who don't eat meat are directed to the side dishes, which are not very hearty and don't provide balanced nutrition. "What kinds of alternative proteins do you offer for kids who don't eat meat?" Suggest that meats are packaged separately from salads or wraps, so they can be optional add-ins rather than mandatory inclusions—and while they're at it, can they package up some tofu or tempeh? (Some schools are starting to implement plant-based options. Check out www.healthyschoolfood.org for inspiration.)

Bring On the Herbs

There's nothing like fresh basil, chives, cilantro, dill, mint, oregano, parsley, rosemary, and other herbs to punch up the flavor of your plant-based dishes. Cut herbs can be expensive and go bad quickly, so consider growing your own. All it takes is a sunny windowsill. Even if they do not live for too long, it is usually the most economic route to go.

No fresh herbs in the house? Keep a stock of dried herbs, replenishing them regularly for the most vibrant flavor. (Note: Chives, dill, and parsley don't translate very well when dried—these are best used fresh.) If you have access to a store that sells bulk dried herbs, you can buy them in small batches for less waste.

Grab-and-Go Options

The world is definitely starting to catch up with plant-based eating on the road. Make it easier on yourself by having some of these quick options on hand. Here's a mix of homemade and prepared foods that you can grab in no time:

MAKE AT HOME:

- Apple, pear, or other fruit spread with nut butter
- Celery or carrot sticks spread with nut butter or hummus
- Romaine leaf filled with hummus
- Whole grain crackers with almond butter and jam
- Whole grain noodles tossed with white beans, chopped fresh tomato, and basil
- Chai soy latte (chai tea bag steeped in hot soy milk)
- Tortilla with mashed avocado and salsa
- Avocado toast—plain or with tomatoes
- Mashed canned beans with olive oil and herbs
- Toast squares with vegan cream cheese and sliced cherry tomatoes, salt, and pepper on top
- Bagel with vegan cream cheese with sugar-free preserves, cut in little pieces for sharing
- Shake (plant-based milk or yogurt, ripe banana, other fruit; see pages 201–203 for Jasper's recipes)

- Mug with a few tablespoons of granola and plant-based milk
- Dried figs stuffed with almond butter
- Whole wheat pita bread dipped in olive oil with za'atar or spread with tapenade
- Rice cake with vegan cream cheese and bell pepper
- Tortilla with melted vegan cheese and sliced tomato
- Sautéed tempeh strips dipped in Jasper's Peanut Sauce (see page 259, or use jarred peanut butter dipping sauce)
- Frozen veggie burger (with a mushroom-, bean-, quinoa-, or other whole-food base)

PREPARED (FROZEN, TAKEOUT), BUT YOU COULD ALSO MAKE THESE YOURSELF:

- Frozen plant-based pizza (or homemade with Miyoko's Creamery vegan cheese and pizza sauce)
- Small bean burrito
- Avocado and cucumber sushi roll
- Steamed edamame with salt
- Soy nuts
- Chickpea snacks (roasted chickpeas–store-bought, or make at home)
- Trail mix (store-bought, or make at home: 3 parts almonds, 2 parts walnuts, and 1 part golden raisins or half golden raisins and half dried apricots)
- Cup of instant black bean or lentil soup
- Miso soup with tofu
- Soy latte
- Fruit-and-nut bar or other plant-based energy bar (like KIND bars)
- Plant-based yogurt (soy, almond, cashew)
- Seaweed snacks

Add Some Umami

In addition to sweet, sour, bitter, and salty, we can sense a fifth taste—umami. This taste gives food complexity and richness—but unfortunately, it's mostly found in animal products like meat, cheese, and fish. To head off any umami cravings as you cut out meat, add in some plant-based sources right at the start. Good sources include meat alternatives (like Beyond Meat or Impossible Foods burgers), fermented foods (sauerkraut, kimchi, soy sauce, liquid aminos, balsamic vinegar, and tempeh), kelp, shiitake and porcini mushrooms, ketchup, and toasted seeds and nuts. Also wonderful is nutritional yeast, the plant-based eater's best friend (see "Grab the Nooch," below).

GRAB THE NOOCH

When I went plant-based, one other thing I did crave, in addition to the cream in my tea, was cheese—I would eat spoonfuls of plant-based "cheese" shreds after dinner. Then I found nutritional yeast, and I sprinkled it on everything.

Nutritional yeast is a deactivated yeast that, contrary to popular belief, does not always contain B_{12}, so you have to check. "Nooch" (as it's affectionately known) is a great supplement to many recipes, packing 9 grams of complete protein per serving and bringing in a nutty, creamy note that reminds many of cheese. You can sprinkle it on popcorn and pasta, in soups and sauces—nooch adds body, complexity, and that umami flavor that you may be missing without cheese.

One night, I had just opened a new bag of nooch, and I ate 5 tablespoons—I guess you could say I had a little problem at that point. Well, about ten minutes later, Rose came over and she said, "Mommy, your face is all red—you've got spots all over your knuckles." She was right. My wrists were red, my knees and ankles were red. I ran into the bathroom and had a really blotchy face–my ears were tingling and hot. What the heck??

Turns out that nooch has a really high level of niacin–so I was having what's known as a "niacin flush." (When you take too much niacin, the small blood vessels in your face dilate so much that your skin turns red.) So now when I have nooch, I stick to one spoonful.

What's the True Cost?

We are constantly encouraged to eat the food the government subsidizes because those foods are artificially priced to be more affordable. Check out the distribution of USDA and other industry subsidies from the government:

Meat and dairy: 63%
Grains: 20%
Sugar: 15%
Nuts and legumes: 2%
Fruits and vegetables: 1%

Up That Produce Ratio

Up until now, I've focused a lot on how we replace animal proteins with plant-based alternatives. That's because when we make this transition, we tend to focus our attention on compensating for what's not there anymore. For me, the true magic and beauty of plant-based eating has always been what *is* there instead: the rainbow of fruits and vegetables. When you subtract the animal foods, thousands of new vegetables, fruits, nuts, seeds, legumes, and whole grains now move to the center of the plate. The possibilities are endless!

How OMD Helps the Earth

In 2016, the World Resources Institute did a study looking at how steady transition to more plant-based eating could help the earth. They analyzed six different scenarios, and here's what they found:

Eating Pattern	If you ...	You will ...
Ambitious animal protein reduction	Eat half as much meat, dairy, eggs, and fish as you do now.	Protect 45% more land. Produce 43% less greenhouse gas from food.

If everyone did it, we'd save ... A land mass twice the size of India.
And we'd eliminate ... Three times the *total* greenhouse emissions from 2009.

Traditional Mediterranean diet	Eat more fruits, vegetables, pulses, whole grains, fish, and poultry; and eat less red meat, sugar, and full-fat dairy.	Protect 11% more land. Produce 11% less greenhouse gas from food.
Vegetarian diet	Eat more fruits, vegetables, pulses, whole grains; eat no meat or fish; eat less full fat dairy and eggs.	Protect 48% more land. Produce 56% less greenhouse gas from food.
Ambitious beef reduction	Eat 70% less beef than you do now.	Protect 33% more land. Produce 35% less greenhouse gas from food.

If everyone did it, we'd save ... A land mass the size of India.
And we'd eliminate ... Twice the *total* greenhouse emissions from 2009.

Shift from beef to pork and poultry	Eat 33% less beef and replace it with pork and poultry.	Protect 13% more land. Produce 14% less greenhouse gas from food.
Shift from beef to legumes	Eat 33% less beef and replace it with beans and soy.	Protect 15% more land. Produce 16% less greenhouse gas from food.

I want to encourage you to think of yourself as a little kid and this transition to plant-based eating as an unlimited playdate. Relearning how to cook as a plant-based eater is a never-ending experiment, an ongoing art project, an investigation into your own preferences and palate. Plant-based eating is simply gorgeous—slice into a kiwi and notice the pattern of the seeds. Marvel at the blue-green of a fresh head of broccoli. Take a moment to revel in the kaleidoscope of colors in the fruit aisle. (Contrast that with the vision of raw chicken or pork sitting on the counter—not as appetizing!) Have fun with the recipes in chapter 7—get your whole family involved in selecting the produce, hunting down new grocery items, prepping and cooking in this new way, and taking pictures. These new creations are mini masterpieces that you get to eat—and feel really good about. Please come to https://www.facebook.com/OMD4thePlanet/ and share them with us!

Perhaps one of the best benefits? You never have that food-hangover moment of "Ugh, I shouldn't have eaten that" when you're on a plant-based diet. Even the most decadent chocolate mousse (see page 278) is ultra-nourishing and feeds your body on a cellular level. Here are a few suggestions of how to punch up the produce ratio during your transition.

Start with a veggie tray or a big salad. One trick I've learned is that kids will eat whatever you give them when they're hungry. So while the main dish is cooking, I'll put out a gigantic platter of cut veggies (cucumbers, carrots, cherry tomatoes, etc.) and a bunch of small dishes of dipping sauces (guacamole, hummus, vegan ranch dressing). While they're eagerly waiting for dinner, they chomp away at the veggies, and I feel like half my nutritional responsibility is fulfilled before the casserole dish even hits the table.

Another favorite: a big Caesar salad. I don't know how often I've put that out and the kids come back for seconds before they even eat their main course. If they're hungry, they will eat that first.

This works especially well if you get them in the habit when they're younger!

Go on a color hunt. Going to the farmers' market with the kids is so much fun. I admit—we are spoiled in California. You can find vegetables that you don't see in grocery stores, like purple broccoli or purple cauliflower. At peak season, one stall at the market might have sixteen different varieties of plums. During the fall, I love to see how many different shades of carrots we can find, then put out a carrot rainbow for dipping. Quinn loves to make mashed potatoes, and this past summer we made mashed purple potatoes—yum.

Build on a veggie base. Make veggies the foundation, then layer on top of them. For example, cut a roasted or cooked sweet potato in half and pile on a bunch of roasted or sautéed vegetables. Cook up some spaghetti squash and load on some Bolognese sauce (see page 246). Try using a spiral slicer to make "noodles" from zucchini. (See Melissa's Coodle Cups with Dill-icious Mango Sauce on page 219 for a fun way to do this.)

Create a Mexican fiesta. Over the summer, when the kids and I all have a lot more flexibility in our schedules, we rotate the dinner duty from beginning to end. Each kid has their dinner, and they do everything: shop with me, plan the meal, prep all the ingredients, and cook the food, and then we sit down to eat and share the whole experience.

"Mexican fiesta" is Quinn's go-to. He has a killer guacamole recipe (see page 254), and he chops all the veggies and puts them out in dishes, with sauces, taco shells, and tortillas so we can all make our own tacos and burritos. We create a taco bar using Ree Ree's Raw Vegan Taco Nut "Meat" (page 226) and Pagie Poo's "Cazzewww" Cream (page 257), so named because Mom calls cashews "cazzewwws."

How to Soak Beans

Beans are an incredibly healthy and versatile food, whether they're canned or soaked and cooked from scratch. If you're buying canned, look for BPA-free cans or cartons, and get them either salt-free or low in sodium (under 150 mg per ½ cup).

As handy as canned beans are, I want to put in a big plug for dried beans. First of all, they're inexpensive! You can get a ten-pound bag of organic black beans, the equivalent of forty cans of beans, for about twenty bucks at Walmart. Considering a can of organic black beans is usually around $2 to $3, that's a huge savings. Cooked dried beans taste better, can be firmer (if you need them to be), and give you complete control over sodium—and you don't have to worry about chemicals in the canning material.

The overnight soak: Place the beans in the pot you're going to cook them in and add water to cover by at least 2 inches. Leave on the counter—no need to refrigerate—to soak for up to 12 hours. The following day, drain the beans. Add fresh water to cover, bring to a boil, then reduce the heat to maintain a simmer, cover, and cook until tender (about 25 minutes for lentils and up to 2 hours for tougher beans). Soaking overnight cuts down the cooking time (because the beans are softer going into the cooking), and by throwing away the soaking water, you also get rid of some of the compounds beans contain that can make you gassy.

If you forget to soak, no worries! Most beans (especially if they are not old) take from 30 minutes (lentils even less) to 2 hours to cook. Simply rinse them, put them in a pot, cover with a lot of water, bring to a boil, reduce the heat to maintain a simmer, and cook until tender. Or just use your Instant Pot (see "Five Brilliant Instant Pot Hacks" on page 233 for instructions).

Quinn's Pizza Matrix

One of Quinn's specialty dinners is pizza, and he's created the Pizza Matrix to perfect his technique. He puts out all the ingredients, we compose our own personal pizzas, and he cooks them up for us. Here are a few of his favorite combinations, though the possibilities are virtually endless. Bake in a preheated 450°F oven until the nondairy cheese has melted, about 10 minutes.

Crust	Base	Toppings	Plant-Based "Cheese"
Pizza crust	Tomato Sauce	Sautéed peppers, onions, broccoli	Daiya shreds
Tortilla	Refried beans	Corn	Miyoko's Creamery nut cheese
Bagel	Quinn's Pesto (page 260)	Sliced plant-based sausage or Hungry Planet sausage crumbles or Beyond "beefy" crumbles	Follow Your Heart mozzarella shreds

Lay out a pasta bar. Rose loves to make pasta—in the height of summer, we all love eating her homemade tomato sauce. We'll do a pasta night with three kinds of pasta—penne, fusilli, and spaghetti—and then three kinds of sauce—Quinn's pesto, Rose's tomato sauce, and a Bolognese—and everyone gets three little bowls to customize their own sampler.

Let them get their chef on. I love just hanging out in the kitchen sometimes and watching to see what the kids will come up with when they get hungry. One summer, Rose had a friend over for a sleepover, and she offered her pal some salad. She went out back to the garden, got some tomatoes and herbs, brought them back into the kitchen, and set to work, chopping away with her gigantic chef's knife like she owned the place. Another morning, I offered her some pancakes, and she said, "No, Mom—I'm going to have garden breakfast." She headed out to the garden and came back in with a huge cucumber in one hand and a tomato in the other, alternating big bites from each while their juices dripped copiously down her arms, face, the front of her shirt—a sight that would've made any mother smile. The cutest thing!

Spring roll assembly line. My brother Charlie is famous for his spring rolls—we stole this idea from him and do it all the time together. (Check out the recipe on page 243.) We use rice paper wraps—you dip them in cold water for 5 seconds and then fill them with fresh vegetables, sprouts, and mint, and top them with Jasper's Peanut Sauce (page 259). This dinner is one of the best crowd-pleasers, because everyone can make their own meal exactly the way they want to. Huge hit with all the kids and their friends.

Ben's Afternoon Tea. One of my very favorite snacks that Ben ever made was a twelve-course afternoon tea with Rose and one of her friends—every single course was a little nibble made from vegetables or fruits. He made savory bites like small round rice cakes with vegan cream cheese and half a cherry tomato on top, with a sprinkle of salt and pepper, and sweet ones, like PB&J cut into small animal shapes using cookie cutters. Another day, he made a veggie chess set—he wove a mat from palm fronds that was so beautiful and colorful, and used these (in fun combinations) to make the chess pieces:

 apple
 banana
 clementine
 avocado
 strawberries
 cashews
 peach

This was early in our plant-based transition, and by making the afternoon snack into a game, he helped Rose fall in love with this new way of eating. (See photos of the chess set and other fun plant-based activities with the kids at https://omdfortheplanet.com/media-center/gallery.)

Start off sweet. When I serve fruit in the morning, I always give my kids a toothpick to eat it with, and they love it—they're more inclined to eat their bowl of fruit with a toothpick or fancy cocktail pick or fork than with a regular fork.

MY OMD STORY

Zoe Nachum

I'm in seventh grade, and I started to eat plant-based in February 2016. My mom explained to me what happened in slaughterhouses, and I just thought about it a little, then I slowly made a transition. At first, I missed some things that I used to eat, like chicken and cheese, but then I found options that are similar so it started getting easier. I really like soy chicken or tofu. My mom makes it in the same mini-oven on the counter where she used to make the real chicken or other meat. I like the Follow Your Heart American Cheese Slices—I don't eat them a lot, but when I'm craving cheese they're really good. When I first started, I would still eat eggs in cakes or bread. Later on, my mom found an option for bread that doesn't have any eggs: Dave's Killer Bread, which is so good.

On Tuesdays, my old school would get a taco truck. I couldn't get anything because things that didn't have meat had dairy. I had to bring a sandwich from home. I like how at MUSE there's a variety of foods to pick from, with different options every day—I'm not just stuck with one thing. I really like the miso soup! I also like the bowls with rice, onions, and tofu. We go down the food counter line and we pick different veggies to add to our bowls.

If someone my age is thinking about going plant-based, I suggest they do their research. Maybe they could look into what kinds of foods are plant-based and which aren't, or what happens inside of a slaughterhouse or a dairy farm. Learning about that really touched my heart and helped me make this decision. And eating meat and dairy is so bad for the environment too. I would tell kids to try it—maybe they'll like it!

Pro Tips

A little underconfident in the kitchen? No worries. Here are a few easy rules of thumb to help prepare veggies when you're new to OMD.

Cut all your veggies the same size. Not that you have to get it right to the millimeter, but if you slice and chop vegetables to be reasonably uniform, they will cook that way, meaning your broccoli, potatoes, or other vegetables will have about the same level of bite, crunch, or softness throughout the dish.

Dice for speed. In a hurry? The smaller you slice or chop or dice them, the quicker your vegetables will cook. This is especially dramatic for vegetables that take ages to cook, such as beets and potatoes. A grated (or very thinly sliced) sweet potato can cook in a 400°F oven in 10 to 15 minutes versus 45 minutes for a whole sweet potato.

Grate sweet potato or beets into soup. This gives the soup extra body that makes it feel super hearty. If you don't have time to grate, you can buy pre-shredded veggies at most grocery stores.

Grate veggies into your salad . . . and then squeeze an orange over the top so the vegetables don't brown. One of my favorite staples in Paris was the *salade de crudités*—grated carrots, beets, and zucchini drizzled with a simple little vinaigrette. So good, I can still remember the first time I ate one.

"Quesa"-dillas and breakfast burritos. My kids have always loved quesadillas. We went from cheese quesadillas with a little bit of vegetables in them to lots of sautéed vegetables with a little bit of vegan cheese and refried beans. Claire's favorite is to mix a can of refried pinto beans with a can of black beans and use that mixture in a burrito. (And, again, be careful with the vegan cheese—some are really good, but some of them, not so much. See page 295 for my recommendations.)

I used to make breakfast burritos that had beans and salsa, and I would put scrambled eggs in them. Now we make them with tofu scramble, pinto beans, and black beans, and we sauté whatever kinds of vegetables we have in the crisper and top it all with salsa. The whole family loves it.

Hobo dinners. We had an old cast-iron bathtub that's been outside our Colorado house forever, and the kids loved to use it to build a fire and make some s'mores (with vegan marshmallows). One night, the kids said, "We should make hobo dinners!" a fun meal I learned how to make at camp. So we found some heavy-duty foil, put in some white and sweet potatoes, Beyond Meat "beefy" crumbles, onions, red bell peppers, garlic, squash, and Daiya cheese, and wrapped everything up. Once the fire burned down to coals, we threw the hobo dinners on and let them cook. Then we all sampled one another's concoctions. This is also a great thing to do inside in your fireplace on a long winter's night. You can also cook corn on the cob or even bake an apple cobbler this way.

HOW DO YOU GET YOUR KIDS TO EAT VEGETABLES?

I have this friend who was always incredulous when she came to my house: "Oh my goodness, how do you get your kids to eat vegetables?" She said her daughter would only eat doughnuts and pizza. "That's all she'll eat, so that's all we give her."

I suggested she start out easy. Put out some dipping sauces and cut up a cucumber. Just say, "Let's try this vegetable tonight. Just try it, and then you can have a slice of pizza." Within a few weeks, her girls were both trying new vegetables every night.

Another way to engage them with eating more plants is to help them to grow their own vegetables. You don't need a yard—you can grow cherry tomatoes in a planter on a balcony or back patio, or even in a bunch of pots on the windowsill. If your child can see things growing and eat them right off the vine or out of the dirt, there's no better way to get them intrigued. You could even work up to a community garden.

We have to believe that kids will challenge themselves if we trust them. And if all else fails, the old parenting rule applies: if they're hungry enough, they will eat.

Yup—We Are Vegan, and We Raise Bees

Strict ethical vegans do not eat honey. We do—in fact, we raise our own bees, so we know our honey is responsibly and ethically sourced. And we have very happy bees.

Every year, we increase our bee population at our home in New Zealand by one-third. We started with 100 hives and now have 450. We also sell our excess hives to neighbors, so we can all help support the pollinator population in New Zealand.

In the States, we don't have hives, but we plant tons of pollinator bushes and ice plants in the garden, so bees are constantly swarming around. In fact, when the ice plants' flowers are open, we've learned to be very gentle near the plants—the slightest knock could spook an entire cloud of bees out of hiding. Feels good to know we're helping boost the dwindling population of honeybees on both sides of the world—and getting yummy honey to boot. If you eat honey and want to make sure what you buy is ethically sourced, buy honey from local individual beekeepers who practice "balanced beekeeping" and/or look for a "True Source Certified" label on the jar. Also, buy in small batches, and only use honey as a treat instead of a staple.

The 14-Day OMD Transition Plan

I f you'd like a more structured way of trying OMD, look no further. I've picked a range of OMD recipes to show you how easy this can be. These weekday recipes are all versatile and many lend themselves to other recipes, so you can use leftovers to build another OMD meal plan. Plus, they're super fast and generally easy to make ahead.

DAY 1: MUSE-li Mix (page 204)

Start your day with a delicious bowl of MUSE-li, the perfect make-ahead breakfast. Combine 1 cup of the dry MUSE-li Mix with about a quarter of an apple, coarsely grated, and about ¼ cup almond milk. Top with fresh fruit as desired.

TIP: Almond milk isn't just for MUSE-li—you can use it on all your favorite cereals to make them instantly OMD-friendly.

DAY 2: Basic Black Beans (page 224)

Canned beans make this recipe quick work; you can use these black beans in just about anything, from your morning breakfast burritos to a simple dinner of rice and beans.

TIP: Instead of using premade canned refried beans, which often contain animal fats, whirl up these beans in a food processor instead. Add a little tomato juice if you prefer a thinner consistency.

DAY 3: Ree Ree's Cheese Spread (page 255)

This protein-packed spread is super satisfying when you're craving something cheesy. Plus, it's super easy to put together. Spread it on whole grain toast and top with tomatoes and cucumbers for a quick lunch option.

TIP: This dish does double-duty as a great snack served on top of crackers or with fresh vegetables for dipping; consider making a double batch, as it will keep well in the fridge for about a week.

DAY 4: BBQ "Chicken" Sliders with Classic Coleslaw (page 236)

We love Beyond Meat frozen "chicken" strips because they're always an easy grab-and-go option for a quick meal. Making some slaw with a bag of pre-shredded cabbage also cuts down prep time considerably. And as for vegan mayonnaise in place of the regular stuff? We promise you won't notice any difference. (See page 295 for a list of our favorite plant-based brands.)

DAY 5: Pagie Poo's Chocolate Mousse (page 278)

You can whip up a batch of this decadent chocolate mousse in less than 10 minutes. Let it chill in the fridge and you'll have a company-worthy treat on hand at a moment's notice—though it's so rich and satisfying you might want to keep it all to yourself.

TIP: For a whipped tofu dish like this, wrap the tofu in cheesecloth or paper towels and gently squeeze out the excess moisture.

DAY 6: Scrambled Tofu (page 205)

Plant-based proteins can make for a very satisfying breakfast. Make a double batch to have some on hand for an extra-quick meal in the morning.

TIP: Take a tip from Ben and sauté any veggies you have in the crisper, then wrap them up in a big flour tortilla with the scramble like my kids love to do.

DAY 7: Jasper's Peanut Sauce (page 259)

When you're in the mood for Chinese or Thai food, this sauce will come in handy. Use it as a tasty dip, toss it into some noodles, or consider how it might add an interesting twist to a veggie-loaded sandwich.

DAY 8: Ree Ree's Raw Vegan Taco Nut "Meat" (page 226)

Who doesn't need to satisfy a taco craving now and then? The best part of a recipe like this is that the taco "meat" is made from a mix of nuts and sun-dried tomatoes and comes together in far less time than it takes to brown a pound of hamburger. However, we do recommend that you make a batch early in the morning and refrigerate it; the flavors improve after 6 to 12 hours.

TIP: Why stop with tacos? This nut "meat" is also delicious sprinkled over a Southwestern salad, loaded into a quesadilla, or mixed with some cooked brown rice for an easy side dish.

DAY 9: Lemon-Blueberry-Coconut Scones (page 211)

These scones call for a flax egg, a mixture of ground flaxseed and water that takes the place of a traditional egg in this recipe. In fact, you can use flax eggs to replace chicken eggs in many baking recipes, although it may take some experimenting.

TIP: Ground flaxseed can go rancid quickly, so better to grind just what you need and use it up, or store it in the freezer until you're ready to use it.

DAY 10: Mom Amis's Creamed Corn (page 231)

Sweet, creamy, decadent comfort food—you'll definitely surprise your friends and family when you tell them this is a vegan recipe.

TIP: When corn is in peak season, plan ahead and freeze some extra for this dish—if you'll be cooking the corn in a dish like this, there's no need to blanch it beforehand. Simply cut the raw kernels off the cob, scrape the "milk" from the cob, and load the corn into quart-size freezer bags. Use a straw to eliminate as much air from the bag as possible and enjoy within 2 to 3 months.

DAY 11: Fantastic Falafel (page 222)

Try making your own falafel on a weekend when you have a little more time and can get the whole family involved in assembling their own sandwiches.

TIP: Using canned chickpeas is not just convenient–if you save the liquid from the can, you can use it on day 12 to whip up some sweet meringue cookies for the week ahead.

DAY 12: Saranne's Meringues (page 273)

These sweet treats are traditionally made with egg whites, but you can achieve the same delicious results using the liquid drained from a can of chickpeas. Known as aquafaba, it becomes remarkably light and fluffy when whipped.

DAY 13: Pagie Poo's "Cazzewww" Cream (page 257)

This cashew cream, which essentially is raw cashews soaked in water and then pureed, becomes the basis for many delicious dishes; you can basically use this stuff as you would heavy cream or half-and-half in everything from soups to salad dressings.

TIP: For sweet dishes, omit the garlic, lemon, and nutritional yeast from the recipe and whirl in 3 or 4 pitted Medjool dates in their place.

DAY 14: Spaghetti Bolognese (page 246)

This recipe goes to show that just because you are eating plant-based doesn't mean you have to give up on hearty, satisfying meals. If you like, stir ½ cup of Pagie Poo's "Cazzewww" Cream (page 257) into the sauce for an added boost of flavor.

When You Want to Step It Up

Once you've been doing OMD for a few weeks, stop and check in with yourself—how does it feel? Focus on the positive. What's working the best? Study that success, and duplicate it. If you're enjoying it and you want to start expanding plant-based eating into other meals, you can begin to double your OMDs to two a day—or even more! Or you could try Kathy Freston's approach—designate one day to be AMD (all meals a day). Then *lean* into it, adding another, and another. Here are a few suggestions to add more plant-based meals to your life.

1. Is there a standard meal you enjoy that you could easily eat every day? Many people do plant-based breakfasts: oatmeal with flax milk, cereal with soy milk, tofu scramble. Your OMD is set—no need to think twice. Now start to develop a standard repertoire of lunches in the same way.

2. Challenge everyone in the house to a Green Eater Meter contest— who can save the most gallons of water by the end of the week? Look at your Green Eater Meter tally sheets for this past week. How do they compare to the way you were eating when you started OMD? How many gallons of water have you saved? How many air-choking miles have you spared our poor climate? How many square meters of pristine land have you protected?

3. Eat your way up the Greenhouse Gas Emissions chart in chapter 4. Start with the food that would normally be the focus of your meal (beef or pork) and then move one tick up on the scale (pork or chicken). Keep going and challenge yourself to get to smaller and smaller numbers.

4. Go through chapter 7's recipes and flag six that seem really tasty to you. Commit to eating those in the next week. Take notes, reflect, and repeat the process, adding a recipe a week.

5. Try Meatless Mondays. Or the Reducetarian approach. Or VB6 (vegan before six), Mark Bittman's approach. Whatever speaks to you, your rhythms, your life.

6. Have everyone pick a meal a week that they prepare. Take them shopping, help them meal plan, and be their prep cook (and sous chef, if needed). Helping will up their buy-in and take some of the persuasion pressure off you.

7. Stick with OMD for a month and then, on a specific date, add another meal—and repeat. Then add another meal.

8. And there's always the 21-day challenge—go fully plant-based for 21 days, just to see how it feels. Then, on day 22, add back some animal products and see how you feel. I predict enormous changes. Some people eat some animal products and realize they're not ready to go fully plant-based—but they find they're satisfied with way less meat than before. That's OK!

Give Yourself a Standing O(MD)

How do you feel? Like a freaking rock star, I hope!! You are saving the planet one meal at a time, my friend. You are actively making the world a better place.

If you choose to stick with OMD for the rest of your life, that one switch will be a greater contribution toward the reversal of climate change than anything else you've done in your life. I hope you understand how meaningful that is—it is a tremendous accomplishment. Please share that sense of accomplishment with your friends and your family—tell them how proud you are, and how good you feel, body and soul. Ask them if they would like to join you.

OMD has restored my hope that one individual *can* make a difference, and that together, we have the power to tackle climate change, starting right here, right now. In addition to all the water, greenhouse gases, and land my family has saved since going plant-based, I think about all the other people we've talked to, and I envision the OMD ripple effect in action.

We've turned so many friends, family, acquaintances, parents, teachers, even students on to this way of eating—and how many people have they told? A couple from Australia visited us in New Zealand for two days; afterward, I sent them off with a bag, and now they've been plant-based for three years, maybe four. I bumped into the husband recently. He had always been very quiet and I don't remember him smiling a lot—well, he's dropped thirty or forty pounds, and he's Mr. Smiley-Talky. Another born-again plant-based person, Bill Foley, who grew up on a Texas cattle ranch, walked away from a meeting with us about something totally unrelated with a bag of books and DVDs. After not hearing from him for ten months, he checked in and told us he'd lost thirty-five pounds and taken 100 points off his cholesterol, and his blood pressure had gone from 155/110 to 120/80—all in ten months. His doctor couldn't believe it.

I have dozens of stories like this.

Now, if you're feeling emboldened and inspired, and you take it to the next level, let's talk about All-In—what it takes, how it feels, and all the tremendous health benefits you and your whole family will reap when you make that extra level of commitment to the earth—and to your own life.

chapter 6

All-In

What do you think—are you ready?

APATT! All plants, all the time!

Sometimes there's just a moment in our lives when we want to take a big step toward what's next. Maybe you've done OMD for a few weeks, and you're starting to feel more energy and see more glow in your skin—and you want to go further. Maybe you're feeling sharper than you've felt in years—and you want to see if eating less meat would help even more.

Maybe you've had a recent health scare, and you're ready to make a big shift to change your body's trajectory.

Maybe you're sick of fighting with the scale, and you want an eating approach that's guaranteed, simple to understand and follow, and sustainable for the rest of your life.

Maybe you're sick of seeing the planet in such pain, and you want to do something, anything, to help protect the earth for all the children of the future.

Maybe you've been toying with the idea of going fully plant-based for a while. Or maybe reading this book has given you a lot to think about.

That simple, elegant solution. That one linchpin choice that impacts all others.

You can take control of your life, your family's life, their health, and their future. You. You have the power to change the world.

You don't have to put solar panels on the roof. You don't have to drive an electric car. You don't have to change every single light bulb. Sure, it's great to do all those things too. But if you just pay attention to what kind of food you're buying for your family, and what you're preparing at nighttime, or for lunches, or whatever, that act alone is going to make a huge difference.

You don't have to be perfect. You don't have to turn into a Prius-driving, drum-circle-attending, peace love dove beads bells and incense shaggy-haired hippie tree hugger. Do this, and you basically get a free pass. (Well, maybe don't run out to get a massive gas-guzzling SUV or anything—in a way, meat is the new SUV!)

I'll give you an example: I love taking baths. But I don't take them very often because they use so much water—so when I do, I take it with full awareness, a clear conscience, and I do my best to really, really enjoy them. One night, I was doing my regular debate about whether or not I should take one. Jim came in and said, "Babe. Take the bath. Do you know how much water you saved just at dinner tonight?"

And time. Eating plant-based has begun to create hours of my life that never would have existed before. A Mayo Clinic study published in the *Journal of the American Osteopathic Association* in 2016 determined that seventeen years of eating as a vegetarian can lengthen your life by almost four years (3.6 years, to be exact).[1]

So I did a little calculation: If I pledge to go fully plant-based for the next 17 years, when that 17 years is up, I'll have 3.6 years of bonus life to play with. If I amortize that 3.6 years over every one of the 18,615 plant-based meals I'll eat in those 17 years, it averages out to 101.64 minutes of extra life per meal.

Over an hour and a half more time on earth for each of those delicious, nourishing, energizing meals? Count me in. That is a heck of a deal.

Now, before anyone flips out: I know this calculation isn't even remotely scientifically sound. Lots of mitigating factors here. But as a general guideline, a rule of thumb, a way of quantifying my plant-based journey? I'm going to take the spirit of that fuzzy math on faith.

Going All-In changed every single aspect of my life, in all the best ways. My health improved. I got stronger. My relationships deepened. I became more hopeful for the future. And I embraced a bold and fierce protectiveness for this earth and every living thing on it.

All-In was my vehicle, my path into this new way of being. And, my gosh, it is so deeply fulfilling to help others go All-In too.

The Benefits of Going Big

Every doctor in the OMD brain trust—Dr. Barnard, Dr. Esselstyn, Dr. Campbell, Dr. McDougall, Dr. Ornish—has seen astonishing health transformations in their patients in just a week or two of eating plant-based. Blood pressure dropping 30 points. Cholesterol dropping 50, 70, 100 points. People with arthritis able to walk without pain, or sleep through the night, for the first time in years. People with diabetes drastically reducing, or even going off, their medication.

In just a week or two.

These immediately visible benefits of All-In may help you make the plant-based transition even easier than with OMD. If you've ever tried to manage your cholesterol by cutting out a burger here or there, and had very little to show for it after six months or a year of trying, dropping 50 points from your cholesterol virtually overnight can be a huge turbo boost for your motivation.

You'll see. Since going plant-based, I have way more energy, stamina, and mental and physical energy than I have ever had before. I am in better shape now than I was in my twenties. If you give your body a month, you will be amazed at what happens.

You just have to get through those first few weeks of transition.

Go All-In in Two Jumps

Dr. Barnard advises that people go All-In in two stages. First, take a week to do OMD and check out the possibilities. He advises that you don't change your diet—just take your favorites and tweak them. "Try out the veggie chili instead of the meat chili," he says. "Instead of the meat sauce all over your pasta, try the seared oyster mushrooms or the artichoke hearts." Use cashew yogurt in your smoothie, Earth Balance spread on your toast. Just use your OMDs to try it out.

That week will also give you a sense of how to take your "normal" meals and turn them plant-based. Settle on a few meals that work for you. You'll have a few breakfasts, lunches, and dinners, and maybe a restaurant meal, that you can use as your template.

Once you've been at it for a week or so, the cooking will start to make more sense. "You find recipes and websites and books and all kinds of tools, cool things to buy at the store. You'll discover that a whole lot of other people are doing this too," says Dr. Barnard.

Then he suggests you try All-In for three weeks and see how you feel. "In the same way that when a smoker has quit for three weeks, they feel like a new person. Once you've gotten those gloppy foods out of your diet, after about three weeks, you're feeling better," says Dr. Barnard. "Your blood sugar is better. Your cholesterol is coming down. Your weight's coming down and your tastes are starting to change, and then you've got power you didn't have before."

And then, after three or four weeks, you're there—you're All-In, you're fully plant-based. At that point, if you were to try a double bacon cheeseburger, chances are you would feel very, very sick. "You realize, *I'm just past that*," says Dr. Barnard. "You don't need that anymore."

Changes can be dramatic on All-In—you will likely feel the effects within a few days. You may have a couple of days during which your system reorganizes itself. For those who'd previously eaten a meat-heavy diet, your intestinal flora may struggle a bit to keep up with the task of digesting all this new plant food. You may have a bit of belly discomfort; you may find yourself spending more time in the bathroom than in the recent past. But give it a few weeks—once your system is cleaned out, you will start to feel better than you have in *years*.

MY OMD STORY

Elle Totorici

I used to go to a traditional high school in the Valley. Our cafeteria lunches were so gross, we just brought our own food to school. When I started attending MUSE, I thought, "This is going to be so weird–I'm going to a vegan school." I used to tease my best friend, who's plant-based, that she was missing out on all the good stuff; but, as guest speakers would come to MUSE to talk about plant-based eating and the environment, I started realizing the impact that eating plant-based–or just having one plant-based meal a day–really makes. And, to my surprise, I found I really enjoyed the OMD lunches.

I started watching documentaries, talking to vegans, doing more research. Around the same time, my dad's doctor recommended he try eating plant-based. He asked me to do it with him, and I said yes, of course! So I went raw vegan with him for eighty days.

I wasn't planning to follow a plant-based diet long-term, but then things started to change. I used to get bloated, break out, get rashes, constipated. I was anemic, had hormone imbalances.

Around week two, I thought I had lost a lot of weight because I felt smaller. When I weighed myself, I saw I was the same weight but my bloating had decreased. Then, the acne I'd been battling for years started going away. Compared to the way it was before, now it's nothing. I started feeling super positive about myself and realized, *Gosh, all this has to be from what I'm eating.* The documentaries aren't making stuff up—this is real.

In addition to decreased bloating and acne, I had way more energy. I took a blood test and my white blood cells multiplied! My hormones balanced out and I wasn't having bad periods and all that. Everything just got better and I was completely shocked—I was just doing it for my dad! I didn't think there was anything wrong with *my* health. Eventually, dad ended up going off a medication and lowering his blood pressure too.

Being plant-based is easier than I thought it would be. Even going to restaurants is easy. My friends always say, "Oh, you're vegan—where can we take you?" And I'm like, "Don't worry about me—you guys pick a place; there's always something I can eat."

The hardest part for me in the beginning were the smells. When I first went plant-based and my friends ate pizza or burgers, that was pretty hard. Now, I don't even think those foods smell good. My whole mind has completely shifted. That goes to show how quickly you can break old habits and patterns.

My dad and I made this change basically overnight, but I know the transition is harder for most people. To anyone who wants to try, I would say, it might be tough at first, but take it slow—you can do it!

MY OMD STORY

Sarah Jones

think it's so important that the generation we're raising right now makes better choices than we did. We didn't know we were making bad choices! With OMD, kids learn that you can make your food choices not only for yourself, but also for the environment.

I went vegan about six years ago; my five kids switched about four years ago. My husband made the shift two years ago. Since OMD came to MUSE, I have witnessed an amazing thing: groups of parents who come to MUSE who are not plant-based, then their kids do OMD, and then the parents say, "Oh my god, my child didn't eat anything except steak and french fries before, and now she eats all kinds of vegetables!" The kids see their friends eating that stuff, and they start doing that too. Kids are still learning, so all they do is follow, really. And they say they love the food. Parents that came a few years ago, very skeptical about the plant-based meals, are now turning vegan. The school, and the OMD program, not only makes a shift in the kids, but also a huge shift in the parents.

I cook plant-based at home, but I let the kids eat whatever they want when they're out of the house, at birthday parties, etc. I wanted them to make their own decisions about becoming vegan. My oldest son has a heart condition, so he's always tried to live a really healthy lifestyle. As soon as he heard the data about plant-based eating and heart disease, that was it for him! At MUSE, the students do passion projects, and they're always encouraging them to choose something that will change the world or help make other people conscious. My daughter did hers on veganism—everything she was learning about the animals just struck her heart so much.

But really, there's no wrong reason to choose plant-based—some people just want to look prettier, and that's a good reason too!

Some Mind Tricks for Going All-In

You've read all the proof of how just the singular shift away from red meat can make an enormous difference, both in your own health and the health of the planet. With All-In, the rewards are even greater, but even in All-In, the answer is always "progress over perfection." To that end, here are a few mind tricks that have helped us along the way.

Treat meat like cake. One thing that worked for Jim was that he decided to go all-in, but said from the outset that he would "treat meat like birthday cake"—i.e., have meat once in a while, when he felt like it. Giving himself that out was just what he needed to not feel trapped or afraid that he would fail if he wasn't perfect. So, from May 7, 2012—the day we watched *Forks Over Knives* together—until June 4, 2012, he didn't touch a single animal product.

Then we went away for our anniversary, and he ordered a filet mignon from room service. He saw my raised eyebrow. "What? I told you I wasn't going to be dogmatic about this," he said.

When the food arrived, he dug in eagerly, but about a third of the way in, he got this look on his face like, *Oh, yuck,* and abandoned the filet. For the rest of that day, and the next day, he kept holding his hand over his belly, saying, "Man, I feel like I have a meat hangover."

If you're going to try All-In, but you're a little worried about sticking with it, try the mind trick that Jim used. Tell yourself, "I can have meat anytime I want to. This is not an absolute thing." Giving yourself the out helps you short-circuit any innate rebellion. If you know you're "allowed" to have it any time you want to, you won't feel constrained. All-In will be a choice instead of a mandate.

Reframe the label. One of the biggest frustrations I have is that organic food requires an additional label for what it *doesn't* include, while conventionally raised produce doesn't require a label for what it *does* include—i.e., a ton of chemicals. What if we flipped that?

What if, instead of going to the special organic section, organics became regular "produce," and you had to choose to go to the "chemical produce" section if you wanted conventional stuff? Would that make us a bit more hesitant about picking that food?

If this idea works for you, see how it works for your All-In plant-based transition. Instead of thinking about animal products as the default, think about plant-based food that way. Then the question you ask yourself becomes, *Do I want to eat food—or animals?*

Think pus. Or create your own "eww factor" association to remember when you're feeling tempted. You can always use the funny/scary mind trick that finally did it for my first husband, Jasper's dad, Sam. Sam stayed with us for two weeks during Jasper's wedding celebrations last year, eating plant-based along with us the whole time. He'd been eating mainly plant-based for some time, but during one dinner, he confessed that he was struggling a bit. "Yeah, man, I just have a really hard time cutting out that cream in my coffee."

Jim responded, "Got pus?"

We explained how dairy cows are forced to constantly lactate, which causes frequent (often chronic) mastitis, in which pus is pervasive. The dairy industry fights the high pus count by giving cows antibiotics prophylactically for prevention, not treatment. Imagine the outcry if this was done in human medicine! The massive overuse of antibiotics has led to the emergence of antibiotic resistant superbugs (like MRSA). The loss of effective antibiotics is projected to be one of the major health crises of the twenty-first century.

That was it. Sam hasn't touched milk since. He now says, "All I have to think is 'cup of pus,' and I'm good." (Ewww . . .)

Your All-In Toolkit

et me restate the most important takeaway from OMD: no one is looking for perfection. There is no perfect way to do All-In, just as there is no perfect way to eat, to worship, to work, to play, or to love. You do you, boo. You found a way to incorporate your OMD that worked for you, and that was the right way to do it. You liked getting compliments, because two months after going plant-based, even if you didn't lose a pound, you found that you just glow—you have this beautiful dewy, glowy skin. Sparkling eyes. Thick, shiny hair. And maybe you found you liked the way it feels—and you also take pride in helping to restore the clean air and save those gallons of water, and now you're looking for ways to expand that feeling. To grow the good. That is the perfect way to approach All-In.

That's why we prefer to say "I eat plant-based" instead of saying "I am a vegetarian/vegan." The latter is about a label—and I find it a bit limiting and intimidating. And we are all a little bit rebellious—our first reaction when someone says, "You can't do *X*," is to immediately say, "Hey! Why can't I do *X*?" (Jim had the label maker out recently, and he made a label that read, "I don't believe in labels." I don't like labels, either, except in my fridge and freezer!)

Plant-based is about a choice and an action. I like action. If you'd like a prescribed plan, check out the 14-Day OMD All-In Menu Plan starting on page 187. Personally, I love leftovers (so handy), so you'll notice I've included them throughout. And I've also tried to design the meals in a way that you can use up all the fresh ingredients each week, so there's no wasted food.

Let's do this!

Talk to Your Doctor

Please be sure to talk to your doctor before starting the program, especially if you are under care for a chronic condition like diabetes or heart disease. In talking with Dr. McDougall, Dr. Barnard, and Dr. Ornish, I've heard many stories of people needing to adjust their medication quickly after going plant-based. Granted, many of these people are in residential programs with pretty strict diet plans—but I'm talking, they need to tweak their meds after between 24 and

48 hours on the program. Change happens so quickly. Jim and I didn't have any health conditions, but after three or four days of going plant-based, we looked at each other and said, "Do you feel different?" Happens that fast. So wild.

Fair warning: Your doctor may not be supportive. You may want to bring a book by a doctor, something like *The China Study* or *How Not to Die* or a book by Dr. Neal Barnard. You can also refer them to Dr. Barnard's Physicians Committee for Responsible Medicine website (http://www.pcrm.org/), Dr. Greger's site (http://nutrition facts.org), Dr. Ornish's site (https://www.ornish.com/undo-it/), or Dr. Campbell's site (http://nutritionstudies.org/), or turn them on to the American College of Lifestyle Medicine. If you give it a try, and they don't support you, you might consider finding another doctor. You can find doctors who are supportive of plant-based eating through this great site: https://www.plantbaseddoctors.org/.

I've heard from mothers whose disapproving pediatricians told them that not giving their children cow's milk was child abuse. Do not tolerate that kind of garbage from anyone.

Do Your Kitchen Cleanout

With Jim and me, our first step—literally, the very first thing we did—was to clean out the kitchen. There's something tremendously empowering about physically throwing away the things you're choosing to remove from your life. We had a pile of grass-fed beef, free-range chicken, omega-3-packed eggs, and organic milk and cheese and yogurt. We had goat yogurt from our own goats.

We were so freaked out by this mound sitting on the kitchen counter, it became a philosophical question. We talked about donating it to a homeless shelter—but why would we donate something we believed to be poison? My advice? Give it to your dog or cat or a friend's pet or local animal shelter. Or simply throw it away. There is something very therapeutic and freeing about seeing it in the garbage can. You'll create a visceral connection—not food, garbage. There, done. Our bodies deserve better, and we're not going to treat them like garbage cans anymore.

If this scenario feels wrong to you, I completely understand—I was raised never to waste food, so I truly get that. If that's how you feel, maybe stop buying the products while you're getting ready to go All-In, and when they're gone, that's your moment to start.

Restock Your Pantry

Check out the OMD Master Pantry list on page 295 in the Resource Well (or visit https://omdfortheplanet.com/get-started/resources for a printable version) and take it to the grocery store. You don't have to buy everything at once; you can add products as you go. Just buy enough food for one week, and supplement as you go. Don't forget about dried beans and rice—the cheapest meal in the world and the best foundation for infinite variations.

Prep Ingredients (or Buy Pre-Cut Veggies)

You can put yourself on a good track for the week by prepping some basics on Sunday. Cook several portions of beans and store them, covered, in the fridge (or just have some canned beans on hand). Wash and cut broccoli, cauliflower, zucchini, squash, peppers, carrots, celery—you can grab them for a quick stir-fry or to roast in the oven. Keep a big tub of hummus in the fridge at all times. Buy several bags of lettuce—even one per night—for a dump-and-toss salad. You can prep a few dinners' worth of "chicken" tenders or tempeh at once (see recipe for tempeh on page 189).

Start with Your Favorites

Don't try to go too crazy right out of the gate. We humans are creatures of habit—we all have standard, default dishes in constant rotation. Take the basis of those dishes and construct plant-based versions of them. Once you find a recipe you like, don't feel bad about preparing it again and again. Just get your roster of about two breakfasts, three or four lunches, and four or five dinners—and then cycle through them, adding new meals as you find them. No shame in keeping things simple.

Watch Out for Junk Carbs

Many people are thrilled to welcome pasta, rice, and potatoes back onto the table after many years in low-carb quarantine. All are plant-based crowd-pleasers that you no longer have to avoid (hallelujah!) and all are wonderful transition tools during All-In.

My vices are chips and champagne—Jim and I have our chippies once a week on our date night. I try to buy the healthiest ones I can find, but ultimately, they're still chips. I eat a few corn tortilla chips every night too—unsalted and organic, blue and yellow. They're just so darn good.

That said, as soon as possible, transition away from these "white carbs" to whole grains and sweet potatoes instead. If you give up meat and still eat a bunch of processed carbs, you could run into trouble with your blood sugar. Whole foods are always the way to go.

BE CAREFUL WITH RICE

I drink rice milk every morning, and I eat rice cakes like crazy—I love them both. But we're now finding out about the dangerous levels of arsenic in rice products. (Dr. Greger calls them "arsenic cakes"—sob.) Organic rice still absorbs arsenic from the soil, so that won't protect you, either (double sob). According to *Consumer Reports*, brown basmati rice from California, India, or Pakistan has a third less arsenic than rice from other sources; rice from Arkansas, Louisiana, and Texas has among the highest levels of arsenic.[2] You can reduce the amount of arsenic in your rice by rinsing it, cooking it in a large pot with six times as much water as rice, and then rinsing it again after it's done. The best option, sadly, is to just eat less of it. Other grains—such as amaranth, buckwheat, millet, polenta, bulgur, barley, and farro—have very little arsenic.

Head Off Those Cravings

I'm not going to suggest that going All-In is a piece of cake—it's not. You are detoxing from decades of eating animal products, and the withdrawal can sometimes be tricky. Still, a few strategies can address your cravings and help you get through any initially tough time.

Eat Enough (Good) Fat to Feel Satisfied

The world of plant-based eating has a bit of a philosophical split. Many of our OMD brain trust believe strongly in the Ornish-style, very-low-fat approach (no more than 10 percent of calories from fat). Indeed, Dr. Ornish recommends not adding any fats, oils, avocados, coconut, or olives to your diet. Other plant-based advocates, including the researchers at Loma Linda and Andrews Universities (who helped us create the Green Eater Meter and have done decades of research on vegetarian Seventh-day Adventists in the United States), suggest consuming higher levels of fat, primarily from increased nut intake.

If you're not going plant-based to address a serious health condition, such as heart disease or cancer (and if you are, you should definitely do so under a doctor's care), you don't have to be super dogmatic about your fat intake. To my mind, the most important change here is to feel comfortable, happy, and satisfied while eating a plant-based diet. And plant-based fat definitely helps with that, especially when transitioning off foods that are high in animal fats. Loma Linda researchers have found that eating a daily handful of nuts lowers cholesterol by 10 percent and reduces risk of heart disease by up to 50 percent. No other food has this effect, which is equivalent to that of statins, a class of drugs that lowers the level of cholesterol in the blood by blocking the enzyme in the liver that produces cholesterol. (Another source of cholesterol in the blood is, of course, dietary cholesterol.)[3] Other studies link nuts to lowered risk of cancer, reduced inflammation, and slowed aging process. A recent study also found that nuts strengthen brainwave frequencies linked to thinking, learning, and memory, and others that help us sleep.[4] (Walnuts are the best for this, by the way.)

If sticking with All-In means you eat avocado toast every day, go for it. If it means a handful of nuts carries you through the afternoon, I'm all for it. Many of the most beloved OMD recipes (see chapter 7) feature plenty of nuts and plant-based fat. In the beginning, I ate a lot of cashew nut butter (or crack butter, as my baby brother, Charlie, likes to call it, because it's really that good), pumpkin seed butter, and sunflower seed butter—but I don't anymore. There will likely come a time when you simply crave less fat. I've seen it with Jim, with my kids, and with my extended family. You may find, as you go along, that you don't need as much fat as you do at the beginning—and a little goes a long way. Don't deprive yourself at the start—that sense of deprivation could sabotage your success. Keep your eye on the plant-based prize. You can always tweak as you get more comfortable with plant-based eating in general.

Eat More

Your plant-based meals might require you to eat more to keep up your strength (and avoid belly grumbling) as your digestion becomes more efficient. Just study and pay attention to your digestion rate. If you find your belly grumbling too soon after meals, eat heavier foods. And just eat more plants, period. When I first went plant-based, I felt hungrier, but I just took the opportunity to have a few more servings of my favorite foods. Eat beans or lentils, nut butters, big bowls of oatmeal—odd though it may sound, you can even put some oatmeal in your soup to give it more body. Eat more quinoa, eat hearty grains. Make comfort food, chili. Just don't let yourself get hungry—eating plant-based should be all about pleasure, not deprivation. Jim eats about one and a half times the amount he used to, yet has maintained a thirty-pound weight loss for six years. It works!

Trust Me: Bite the Bullet and Meal Plan

For some people, particularly in busy households with many people running in all directions, meal planning is a lifesaver. For others, meal planning is like scheduling sex—how will I know what I want until that moment?

If you fall into the latter category, I'm going to be super boring and suggest you try to do meal planning, if only for the first few weeks. Meal planning helps you get a sense of your favorite dishes, helps you waste less food, takes some of the pressure off otherwise packed days—heck, it's helpful just to ensure you have the right ingredients in the house so you're not left eating a can of vegetarian baked beans in desperation.

For the no-brainer option, start with the 14-day OMD All-In Menu Plan on page 187. Or print out a meal-planning template at https://omdfortheplanet.com/get-started/resources and plan at least three days at a time. Pick out a few OMD recipes that appeal to you and your eating mates, slot those in, then fill in around them with your simple staple dishes that don't require much work. Double-check what you have in the fridge and pantry, then shop for the rest. Then work the plan, test and tweak, and repeat. Once you discover some favorite plant-based meals, double the recipe next time you cook it and freeze half for an easy weeknight meal.

Meal planning sets you up for success. The longer you do All-In, the easier each part of the process will become—and the more you will start to experiment and have fun with all the variety, the color, the sheer pleasure of plant-based eating.

The 14-Day OMD All-In Menu Plan

Use this handy menu as a guide to plan two weeks of hearty, family-friendly meals. To keep the plan flexible, most breakfast and lunch instructions are written to make one serving (though it's easy to make more), and dinners serve four. An added bonus? When feasible, this plan shows you how to cook ahead and when to save leftovers for easy meals later in the week. (See the 14-Day All-In Menu Plan Shopping List on page 305.)

DAY 1

BREAKFAST: Vegan Sausage Gravy over Toast: To make 1 serving, melt 1 tablespoon vegan buttery spread in a medium skillet over medium heat. Add 1 tablespoon flour, a pinch of salt, and freshly ground black pepper. Cook, stirring until the flour begins to brown, 2 to 3 minutes, then stir in ½ cup unsweetened almond milk and ¼ cup unsweetened nondairy creamer to make a thick gravy. Finely chop 1 or 2 vegan sausages and add them to the gravy. Serve over whole wheat toast.

LUNCH: Vegan Tea Sandwiches: To make 1 serving, spread 2 tablespoons vegan cream cheese over 2 slices whole wheat bread and top with peeled, sliced cucumbers and chopped scallions. Serve with an apple spread with cashew butter alongside.

DINNER: Suzy's Family Favorite Chili (page 230) served with vegan cornbread (made from a mix, with flax eggs, almond milk, and vegan buttery spread in place of animal-based ingredients). Save leftovers for lunch on day 2.

SNACK: Make some popcorn the old-fashioned way on the stove, drizzle with olive oil (instead of butter), and toss with garlic salt and nutritional yeast to taste.

TIP: *To make quick work of your dinner on day 2, bake 4 sweet potatoes while the chili is in the oven. Prick the skins lightly with a fork, rub with a teaspoon of olive oil, and arrange on a baking sheet lined with parchment paper. Bake until soft, about 1 hour.*

DAY 2

BREAKFAST: Easiest Oatmeal: To make 1 serving, combine 1 cup water and ½ cup rolled oats in a 2-cup microwave-safe bowl. Microwave on high for 2 minutes, then stir in 1 tablespoon creamy peanut butter and ½ cup fresh blueberries; drizzle with pure maple syrup, if desired.

LUNCH: Leftover Suzy's Family Favorite Chili

DINNER: Baked sweet potato (see tip from day 1) topped with Garlicky Kale: To make 4 servings of kale, warm 2 tablespoons olive oil in a large skillet over medium-high heat; add 4 chopped garlic cloves, 6 cups chopped stemmed kale leaves, and a dash of red pepper flakes. Cover, reduce the heat to low, and cook for 10 to 15 minutes, until the kale is bright green and tender. Sprinkle with chopped smoked almonds for an added flavor punch, if desired.

SNACK: Really Great Guacamole (page 254) with tortilla chips. Save leftovers for lunch on day 4.

TIP: *To minimize the likelihood that your guacamole turns brown, refrigerate leftovers in a compostable resealable BioBag; squeeze the extra air out of the bag before closing it. To store cut avocados, use the same logic and coat the cut surfaces lightly with olive oil before loading the avocados into the bag.*

DAY 3

BREAKFAST: Chia Pudding: To make 1 serving, begin the night before. Combine 1 cup vanilla coconut yogurt, ½ cup almond milk, 2 tablespoons chia seeds, 1 teaspoon maple syrup, and a pinch of sea salt. Stir, cover, and refrigerate overnight. When ready to serve, top with ½ cup fresh raspberries.

LUNCH: Mexican Wraps: To make 1 wrap, spread 1 large tortilla with leftover Really Great Guacamole, and top with Beyond Meat "chicken" strips, chopped scallions, lettuce, tomatoes, olives, and shredded vegan cheese; roll up like a burrito and serve with chopped fresh mango and bananas.

DINNER: Open-Faced Peppers (page 239) with Jicama Salad (page 241).

SNACK: Enjoy a scoop of your favorite sorbet.

TIP: *To get a jump on your lunch for day 4, in the morning, place an 8-ounce piece of tempeh, 2 tablespoons soy sauce, and ¼ teaspoon garlic powder in a resealable BioBag and refrigerate until you're ready to start dinner. Transfer the tempeh and marinade to a small baking dish and roast in the oven with the Open-Faced Peppers for about 25 minutes, flipping the tempeh halfway through the baking time.*

DAY 4

BREAKFAST: Jasper's Green Shake (page 201) and 1 whole wheat English muffin spread with peanut butter and your favorite jelly.

LUNCH: Tempeh Banh Mi: To make 1 sandwich, spread vegan mayonnaise on a 6- to 8-inch baguette and fill with sliced cooked tempeh (see tip from day 3), sliced radishes, cucumbers, and onion, and top with a spoonful of chopped fresh cilantro. Serve with a small bowl of fresh mango chunks alongside.

DINNER: "Chicken" Fajitas (page 227) served with rice and beans on the side. Be sure to save any leftover vegetables for lunch on day 5.

SNACK: Fruit and Nut Mix: Enjoy your favorite combination of nuts and dried fruit.

DAY 5

BREAKFAST: 1 cup chopped fresh melon topped with ½ cup fresh blueberries, and your favorite vegan breakfast sausage

LUNCH: Southwestern Salad: To make 1 salad, toss 2 cups chopped romaine lettuce with 1 tablespoon olive oil, 1 teaspoon fresh lime juice, and a dash of chili powder. Top with leftover fajita fixings from day 4, as well as any leftover tempeh or radishes you have on hand. If you have any remaining tortilla chips, crumble up a few to add some crunch (instead of croutons).

DINNER: Quinn's Easy-Peasy Pizza (recipe ideas on page 158). This is a very free-form approach to pizza night. Use our chart and your imagination to create your favorite vegan combinations! (Note: Please add your desired ingredients to your shopping list.)

SNACK: Enjoy a nice-size piece of dark chocolate and some fresh raspberries.

DAY 6

BREAKFAST: Decadent Scrambled Tofu: To make 1 serving, crumble
1 (4-ounce) piece of drained firm tofu into large, ragged chunks. Melt
1 tablespoon vegan buttery spread in a small skillet over medium heat.
Add the tofu and sprinkle with a dash each of onion powder, garlic powder,
ground turmeric, and salt. Cook, stirring occasionally, for 2 to 3 minutes,
until the tofu begins to brown. Add up to 3 teaspoons of vegetable broth,
one at a time, until the broth has been absorbed and the tofu is bright
yellow and creamy. Serve with whole wheat toast and fresh strawberries.

LUNCH: Mediterranean Chopped Salad: To make 1 salad, toss 2 cups chopped
romaine lettuce with 1 tablespoon olive oil, 1 teaspoon fresh lemon juice,
and a dash each of salt, pepper, and garlic powder. Top with chickpeas,
olives, and chopped tomatoes, cucumber, and onion. Spoon the salad into
whole wheat pitas, if desired.

DINNER: Brad and Sandy's Sun-Dried Tomato and Asparagus Lasagna (page
250). To complement the rich intensity of this company-worthy dish, serve
it with a mild vegetable, such as cooked yellow squash. And plenty of garlic
bread, of course! Save leftovers for lunch on day 8.

SNACK: Pagie Poo's Lemon Cheesecake Mousse (page 277). Start these
cheesecakes early in the day so the graham cracker crust has plenty of
time to set up. The lemony flavor only improves with time. Save leftovers
for a snack on day 7.

DAY 7

BREAKFAST: Ben's Apple-Walnut "Mouffins" (page 213) and soy or coconut
yogurt topped with fresh strawberries. Save leftover muffins for breakfast
on day 8.

LUNCH: Spinach–Sweet Potato Soup (page 215). Serve with vegan grilled
"cheese" sandwiches (use vegan cheese and butter in place of animal-
based ingredients) and fresh tangerines; save leftover soup for lunch on
day 9.

DINNER: Baked Potato Bar: Bake 6 large russet potatoes in a 350°F oven for 1 hour (see tip). Serve topped with your choice of shredded vegan cheese, salsa, chili, chopped steamed broccoli, chopped onions, and/or vegan sour cream. Save 2 leftover potatoes for the breakfast hash on day 8.

SNACK: Enjoy leftover Pagie Poo's Lemon Cheesecake Mousse from day 6.

TIP: *If you want to avoid turning on your oven, try baking your potatoes in your slow cooker or Instant Pot. If using a slow cooker, prick the potato skins with a fork, drizzle with olive oil, and sprinkle with salt and pepper. Wrap in foil, place in the slow cooker, cover, and cook on Low for 8 hours. If using an Instant Pot, simply prick the potato skins (no need to wrap them in foil), drizzle with olive oil, sprinkle with salt and pepper, and arrange them on the rack insert (make sure the potatoes are all about the same size). Add 1 cup water to the bottom of the pot and carefully follow the manufacturer's directions to seal and cook for 10 minutes on high pressure. Let the pressure release naturally, about 20 minutes, before opening the pot.*

DAY 8

BREAKFAST: Heavenly Hash: To make 1 serving, warm 1 tablespoon olive oil over medium-high heat in a medium skillet. Add 1 chopped leftover baked potato, ¼ cup chopped onion, and ¼ cup chopped bell pepper. Cook, stirring occasionally, for 5 to 7 minutes, until the potato begins to brown and the other vegetables soften. Season with salt and black pepper and scatter 1 tablespoon chopped fresh parsley on top. Serve with leftover Ben's Apple-Walnut "Mouffins" from day 7.

LUNCH: Enjoy leftover lasagna from day 6 alongside a simple Caesar salad: To make 1 serving of salad, use a fork to mix 1 tablespoon vegan mayonnaise and 1 teaspoon fresh lemon juice in a bowl until thoroughly combined. Season with garlic salt and pepper. Add 1 cup chopped romaine lettuce and toss to coat; top with 2 tablespoons crushed vegan croutons.

DINNER: Food Forest Organics Burgers (page 238) with all the fixings. Serve hummus and fresh carrot sticks on the side. To get a jump start on cooking, make an extra 3 cups brown rice for fried rice on day 9; wrap and freeze leftover burgers for lunch on day 14.

SNACK: Enjoy Vegan Banana Splits: To make 1 serving, top a few scoops of your favorite vegan ice cream with sliced bananas, chopped nuts, a drizzle of chocolate sauce, and vegan whipped cream (see tip), if desired.

TIP: *For an extra-indulgent treat for your sundaes, keep a can of coconut cream in the back of your fridge to use for vegan Whipped Coconut Cream (page 274).*

DAY 9

BREAKFAST: Oatmeal with Roasted Peaches (page 207). Serve topped with any leftover Whipped Coconut Cream you might have saved from the sundaes the night before.

LUNCH: Ree Ree's Cheese Spread (page 255) on crackers with leftover Spinach–Sweet Potato Soup from day 7

DINNER: Vegan Fried Rice: To make 4 servings, heat 1 tablespoon toasted sesame oil in a large skillet or wok over high heat. Add 2 minced garlic cloves, 1 tablespoon grated fresh ginger, 1 teaspoon ground turmeric, 1 chopped small carrot, 1 chopped small onion, and 2 cups chopped broccoli. Cook, tossing occasionally, for 3 to 5 minutes, until the vegetables begin to soften. Add 3 cups leftover cooked rice and cook, tossing continuously, until the rice is bright yellow and warmed through. Sprinkle with chopped fresh cilantro and crushed peanuts. Add a dash of sriracha sauce, if desired. Serve with fresh oranges alongside.

SNACK: Enjoy fresh cucumber slices topped with vegan cream cheese, a dash of garlic salt, and fresh finely chopped chives, if desired.

DAY 10

BREAKFAST: Decadent Scrambled Tofu (see instructions on day 6) with whole wheat toast and fresh melon

LUNCH: Mediterranean Wrap Sandwich: To make 1 sandwich, spread a large whole wheat tortilla with hummus, olives, and chopped lettuce, tomato, onion, and cucumber. Serve with fresh grapes alongside.

DINNER: Scooter's Okra and Tomatoes (page 235). Serve over converted white rice with Stewed Collard Greens: To make 4 servings of collards (with leftovers for dinner on day 14), melt 2 tablespoons coconut oil in a large deep pot over medium-high heat. Add 1 chopped large onion and 1 teaspoon red pepper flakes. Cook for 3 to 5 minutes, until the onion softens. Add 1 pound chopped fresh collard greens and 3 cups vegetable broth. Stir until thoroughly combined. Reduce the heat to low, cover, and cook for 35 to 40 minutes, until the collards are very tender.

SNACK: Enjoy fresh strawberries topped with Whipped Coconut Cream (page 274; see tip from day 8).

DAY 11

BREAKFAST: 1 whole wheat English muffin spread with peanut butter and topped with 1 sliced banana and a drizzle of agave syrup

LUNCH: Rio's Marinated Kale Salad (page 218). Serve with 1 apple.

DINNER: Pesto Stuffed Mushrooms: To make 4 servings, stem 4 large portobello mushrooms and scrape out the gills. Rub with olive oil and sprinkle with salt. Arrange the mushrooms rounded side up on a rimmed baking sheet. Roast in a preheated 400°F oven for 10 minutes. Remove from the oven, flip the mushrooms, and fill each with about 1 tablespoon Quinn's Pesto (page 260), 2 tablespoons roasted red pepper strips, 2 tablespoons shredded vegan mozzarella, 1 tablespoon panko bread crumbs, and a light drizzle of olive oil. Roast for 10 minutes more, until softened. Serve each stuffed mushroom on a bed of quinoa, with a side salad of arugula and grape tomatoes tossed with olive oil and balsamic vinegar.

SNACK: Enjoy your favorite crackers with leftover Ree Ree's Cheese Spread from day 9 and a cup of fresh grapes.

DAY 12

BREAKFAST: MUSE-li Mix (page 204) topped with almond milk; serve with 1 small orange alongside.

LUNCH: Eggless "Egg" Salad in Lettuce Cups: To make 1 serving, in a small bowl, mix 2 tablespoons vegan mayonnaise, 1 teaspoon Dijon mustard, 1 teaspoon pickle relish, and a dash of ground turmeric. Stir in ½ (14- or 16-ounce) package chopped drained extra-firm tofu until thoroughly combined. Season with salt and pepper. Spoon the mixture into lettuce cups and serve with carrot sticks and celery.

DINNER: MUSE-y Joes (page 225) served with Roasted Sweet Potato Fries: To make 4 servings of fries, peel 2 large sweet potatoes and slice into long planks. Toss with 2 tablespoons olive oil, 1 tablespoon brown sugar, ½ teaspoon chili powder, and ½ teaspoon salt. Arrange on a baking sheet lined with parchment paper and roast in a preheated 400°F oven for 25 to 30 minutes, until lightly browned.

SNACK: Enjoy your favorite nondairy ice cream dessert, such as Tofutti Cuties.

DAY 13

BREAKFAST: Pancakes with Mixed Berry Syrup (page 208)

LUNCH: Mashed Chickpea Salad Sandwiches with your favorite baked chips on the side. To make 1 sandwich, use a fork to roughly mash ½ cup drained canned chickpeas to a chunky consistency. Add a few tablespoons of finely chopped celery, carrot, and scallion. Stir in a few tablespoons vegan mayonnaise and 1 teaspoon Dijon mustard. Place the chickpea mixture between 2 slices of your favorite bread, along with some lettuce and a few tomato slices, if you like.

DINNER: The King's Shepherd's Pie (page 241). Serve with some good hearty bread and an arugula salad dressed with olive oil and balsamic vinegar.

SNACK: Stewed Cherries with coconut yogurt: To make 1 serving of cherries, combine 1 cup frozen pitted sweet cherries, 1 to 2 tablespoons sugar, 1 tablespoon water, and a dash of ground allspice in a small pot. Cook over medium-low heat, stirring occasionally, for 10 to 15 minutes, until the cherries are thawed and soft. Serve over coconut yogurt.

DAY 14

BREAKFAST: Avocado Toast and fresh raspberries. To make 1 serving of toast, mash 1 ripe avocado, sprinkle with a dash of salt and squeeze of fresh lemon juice, then spread over a toasted slice of your favorite bread. Scatter a few sesame, sunflower, or chia seeds on top for an extra fiber boost.

LUNCH: Leftover Food Forest Organics Burgers from day 8. Serve with fresh watermelon chunks and your favorite canned vegan baked beans alongside.

DINNER: Jackfruit Barbecue with Mom Amis's Creamed Corn (page 231) and leftover Collard Greens (see day 10): To make 4 servings of Jackfruit Barbecue, drain 1 (20-ounce) can brined jackfruit and pat dry. Toss with 2 teaspoons chili powder. Warm 1 tablespoon olive oil in a large skillet over medium heat. Add the jackfruit and cook for 2 to 3 minutes, until the spices are fragrant. Stir in ½ cup of your favorite vegan barbecue sauce, reduce the heat to low, cover, and cook for 30 minutes, or until the jackfruit is tender. Uncover the skillet and cook for 10 minutes more, mashing the jackfruit lightly with a fork to the desired consistency, until most of the liquid has evaporated and the barbecue sauce is thick and sticky.

SNACK: Banana "Ice Cream": To make 1 serving, whirl a chopped frozen banana in your food processor for 2 to 3 minutes, until smooth. For a firmer consistency, transfer to an airtight freezer container and freeze for at least 1 hour before serving.

TIP: *Look for canned jackfruit in the Asian section of your grocery store. Make sure it's brined (not sweetened). When cooked, its texture is remarkably similar to that of pulled pork.*

Invite Them Over. Just Don't Say the "V" Word.

When we first went plant-based, we made the mistake of telling everyone we'd be doing a vegan July 4th party that year. And *so* many people didn't come. In hindsight, we should've said, "We're having a party—we'll have burgers and dogs and corn on the cob, and grilled vegetables, baked beans, and potato salad, all that typical stuff. Please come," and left it at that.

After that experience, we learned our lesson. We had a Christmas party and didn't say a word about plant-based eating. People showed up, and they loved the food. They didn't even think twice about it; they didn't ask. It was just delicious food.

Now when we have dinner parties, we don't tell people what's up beforehand—but it comes up during dinner. When our friend and chef Aaron is helping us for the evening, he'll come out and tell people what he's made, and how much of the food came out of the garden. I swear to you—99.9 percent of the time, people walk away saying, "Man, if I could eat like that every day, I'd be vegan."

Guess what, guys? You can! Brad and Sandy's Sun-Dried Tomato and Asparagus Lasagna (page 250) and Food Forest Organics Coco-Mint Slice (page 279) are huge crowd-pleasers. And interactive meals, such as "Create a Mexican fiesta" (see page 156) or Cheri and Charlie's Spring Rolls (page 243), let everyone make exactly what they like.

This year we had a bunch of folks over for a Memorial Day barbecue; not a "v"-word was uttered, everyone ate plant-based— and everyone was happy. Easy-peasy.

All-In Is a Choice, Not a Mandate

An all-or-nothing approach can be energizing—or it can be very alienating. Jim and I went cold turkey, but that's just how we roll—we tend to make decisions and act very quickly. True to form, I went 0 to 60 and became a born-again vegan. I was on my soapbox as much as I could, telling everybody about it. I said, "Look, it's no problem—all you have to do is just stop." I was like the Nancy Reagan of meat eating: "Just say no."

All the while, I had those cravings for cheese. And I'll admit, every Christmas, I still do crave that cup of English Breakfast tea with some half-and-half.

Pretending those cravings don't exist doesn't help anyone. I ruffled a lot of feathers in that time. All my proselytizing came from a good place—I wanted to save people's lives. And the planet. And all the animals. And the oceans. And, and, and . . . I was to the point where I would see people in stores, debating between two different products, and I'd go up and try to talk them into the plant-based version. (My children were *mortified*.)

In retrospect, I know this approach hurt my cause. In my defense, going plant-based for environmental reasons is a "can't put the toothpaste back in the tube" kind of a thing—I saw, so concretely, the damage we were doing to the planet with what was sitting on our plates, and I couldn't unsee it. I truly think that sadness, that despair, and that feeling of hopelessness is what's behind much of the perfectionism in the militant vegan crowd—we see ourselves as the Cassandras of the coming environmental apocalypse or entrusted with the protection of defenseless animals. Still, counting myself as a reformed born-again vegan, I now see that that approach can be stifling and counterproductive, and I've relaxed. I can even laugh at one of Jim's favorite jokes: "How many vegans does it take to screw in a light bulb?" (Answer: "Doesn't matter—we're better than you.")

As funny as that is, sometimes I fear the vegan mission has been held back by a strident hard-line attitude—and I see it in myself sometimes. We need to acknowledge that in the face of all the public pressure, the industry interest groups, family traditions, habit, inertia, even certain health conditions, coupled with the inescapability of animal products in our culture, going fully plant-based in America can be hard. I read a statistic that about 84 percent of people who go vegan "backslide." That only makes sense if you think about this as an all-or-nothing scenario. The backlash against people who have proclaimed themselves vegan but then decide they want a little animal protein back in their lives can be brutal and unforgiving. Veggie-curious people see that attitude and say, "That's clearly not for me." And then we've lost another potential plant-powered planet protector.

Here's a thought experiment: Imagine our Uncle Billy had smoked for thirty years. He's starting to get that guttural rasp that makes everyone worried about lung cancer. Well, Uncle Billy shows up for a family gathering, and he announces that he's going to try to quit.

How thrilled would we be? Over the moon.

Now, let's say Uncle Billy went a few weeks, maybe even a month—and then he broke down and snuck a drag off his buddy's smoke. Would we turn around and say, "I knew it! I knew you couldn't do it. You're not really committed. You're a *fake* nonsmoker."

No. We would not do that. Because we care about Uncle Billy, and we want him to live. We know he needs encouragement and support, not judgment and shame.

We all need to have that same orientation toward *anyone* who is trying to cut down on their animal consumption—including ourselves. I have said this before and can't emphasize it enough . . . Get an OMD buddy! Start a support group with girlfriends, guyfriends, or try to talk your partner into doing it with you. Jim and I have had so much fun doing this together.

This is a long journey, and it ends with better health for everyone—and the planet. Let's support one another in this transition. Let's have compassion and understanding for the challenges. And most of all, let's encourage one another to celebrate the possibilities and enjoy the journey. To discover all the joy, the vitality, the amazing flavors and satisfaction of plant-based eating. Let's create the world we want to live in every day—so our kids, and their kids, can live here tomorrow.

OMD Recipes

Now for the fun part—let's get cooking! I've collected over
fifty of my favorite recipes from everyone in my world—my kids (and
daughter-in-love), my siblings, my mother (and Jim's), dear friends
and colleagues, the chef from MUSE School—and even shared a few
of my own trademark dishes. These recipes are designed for the home
chef and will appeal to those just transitioning into plant-based eating. You'll find kid-friendly meals, comfort food classics, potluck
favorites, and knock-your-socks-off desserts. (You will love bringing them to parties and tricking people, then basking in the adora-
tion when they find out "*This* is vegan?") We even have an elegant
three-course plant-based meal created especially for this book by
my dear friend Patsy Reddy, the governor-general of New Zealand.

Fresh, seasonal vegetables and fruits can elevate any dish, no
matter how simple. Shop at your local farmers' market or become
a member of a local CSA and get to know the produce offered in
your area. Talk to the farmers—ask them which items they recommend every week. Some farmers' markets are more expensive, some
are less, but the taste and increased nutrition of that produce, as
well as the benefit to your local community, are, to my mind, darn
near priceless. (Go at the end of the farmers' market and you can
usually get amazing deals.) And remember that meat is one of the

most expensive things you can buy at the grocery store, even more so when you factor in the hidden costs (see chapter 3).

Most ingredients are available at standard grocery stores, like Walmart, Albertsons, Safeway, Giant, Kroger, Publix, and Piggly Wiggly. Other items, such as the plant-based cheeses, are available in specialty stores or other high quality foods stores (such as Whole Foods, Sprouts Farmers Market, and Wegmans), yet it's getting easier to find these staples at all grocery stores as consumers demand them. I'm certain we'll see a huge boom within the next few years.

As you go, you'll see the Green Eater Meter score for every recipe that used to include animal products. Calculated with the help of Dr. Alfredo Mejia of Andrews University, this score collects all the environmental savings of your plant-based swaps—all the gallons of water you save, the square feet of forest you protect, and the greenhouse gas emissions you prevent from entering the atmosphere (in the equivalent of miles driven). Some foods save a lot of water; some save a lot of land; some save a lot of emissions. Some save a lot of everything (hello, cheeseburgers!). We wanted to make sure you got "credit" for all your savings, so we rounded the numbers and added up all the data points into one Green Eater Meter score, making it easy for you to see, at a glance, the huge positive impact you're having. Or you can just track one of the data points, like water. Which is great! Whatever approach is the most meaningful and motivational for you, that's the way to calculate your (massive!) environmental savings. Set up a challenge with a friend, your partner, or your kids and see who can save the most in one OMD meal, or in one day. Maybe hang a small dry-erase board on the fridge or kitchen wall as a place to track your cumulative savings (your OMD bank!).

Start small with a few dishes and build up your confidence. Have fun with it. Treat this as a fun exploration. Experiment, play, and enjoy the process. You're about to learn how good plant-based eating can taste—and how amazing it can make you feel.

BREAKFASTS

Green Chocolate Milk Smoothie

YES! Chocolate milk for breakfast is indeed possible while doing OMD. A bit of extra spinach in the mix sneaks in a little added nutrient power.

Makes 2 servings

> *2 cups vanilla almond (or other plant-based) milk*
> *2 teaspoons hempseed*
> *1 tablespoon plus 1 teaspoon unsweetened cocoa powder*
> *1 cup baby spinach*
> *2 teaspoons agave syrup*
> *1 cup ice*

In a blender, combine the almond milk, hempseed, cocoa powder, spinach, agave syrup, and ice. Blend on high speed for 30 seconds, or until frothy and smooth.

Per serving: 145 calories; 5 g fat (.5 g saturated fat); 24 g carbohydrates; 3 g fiber; 3 g protein; 0 mg cholesterol; 165 mg sodium

Swapping out 2 cups dairy milk, you save about:
❀ *2 miles of driving* ❀ *6 square feet of land*
❀ *71 gallons of water*

Jasper's Green Shake

Our son Jasper loves to improvise wonderful shakes and smoothies in the morning, relying on whatever fresh fruits and vegetables he happens to have available that day. Here's a winning formula for putting together your own "green" combination. If you add spirulina—a savory, slightly bitter powder made from a blue-green algae that's rich in protein, vitamins, minerals, carotenoids, and antioxidants—you'll get an extra boost of protein and the smoothie will be a brilliant green, no matter what other ingredients you use.   *Makes 2 servings*

> *1 banana, fresh or frozen*
> *1 cup spinach or stemmed kale leaves*
> *1 cup chopped "green" fruit (such as kiwi, honeydew, pineapple,*
>   *green apple, guava, or grapes)*
> *1 cup ice*
> *1 cup plant-based yogurt (such as Forager Project Cashewgurt*
>   *or Kite Hill almond milk yogurt; optional, to make it*
>   *creamier)*
> *2 tablespoons hempseed (optional)*
> *1 teaspoon spirulina powder (optional)*

In a blender, combine the banana, spinach, "green" fruit of your choice, ice, and the yogurt, hempseed, and spirulina, if using. Blend on high speed for 30 seconds, or until smooth.

Note: *This analysis is based on a smoothie made with banana, spinach, honeydew, and cashew yogurt; nutrition analysis will vary if other ingredients are used.*

Per serving*: 160 calories; .5 g fat (1 g saturated fat); 28 g carbohydrates; 3 g fiber; 4 g protein; 0 mg cholesterol; 28 mg sodium

Swapping out 1 cup dairy yogurt, you save about:
❁ *1 mile of driving* ❁ *3 square feet of land*
❁ *35 gallons of water*

39

Green Eater Meter Score

(for yogurt option

Jasper's Red Shake

Jasper's red shake combinations tend to be sweeter than the green ones, so you might choose to make this version when you're craving a good burst of energy to kick-start your day.

Makes 2 servings

> 1 fresh or frozen banana
>
> 2 cups "red" fruit (such as strawberries, raspberries, blackberries, blueberries, red grapes, peaches, plums, nectarines, mango, or cantaloupe)
>
> 1 cup ice
>
> 1 cup plant-based yogurt (such as Forager Project Cashewgurt or Kite Hill almond milk yogurt; optional, to make it creamier)
>
> 1 tablespoon chia seeds (optional)

In a blender, combine the banana, "red" fruit of your choice, ice, yogurt, and chia seeds, if using. Blend on high speed for 30 seconds, or until smooth.

Nutritional info dependent on fruit selection.

Swapping out 1 cup dairy yogurt, you save about:
❁ *1 mile of driving* ❁ *3 square feet of land*
❁ *35 gallons of water*

(for yogurt option)

39
Green Eater Meter Score

MUSE-li Mix

This MUSE-li mix (a favorite muesli served at MUSE School) can be made in advance and stored in an airtight container in the refrigerator for up to two weeks. Top your bowl with sliced bananas, raspberries, or chia seeds—whatever you like!—as suggested in this recipe.   *Makes 8 servings (8 cups)*

  3 cups rolled oats
  1 cup wheat bran
  2 cups walnuts, chopped
  ½ cup dried apricots, chopped
  1 cup chopped dried figs
  10 dates, pitted and chopped

1. Preheat the oven to 350°F. Line a rimmed baking sheet with parchment paper.
2. Spread the oats and wheat bran evenly over the baking sheet and bake until lightly toasted, 20 minutes.
3. Let the oat mixture cool, then transfer it to a large bowl. Add the walnuts, apricots, figs, and dates and mix until thoroughly combined. Store in an airtight container in the refrigerator for up to 2 weeks.

Per serving: 400 calories; 19 g fat (2 g saturated fat);
56 g carbohydrates; 12 g fiber; 10 g protein;
0 mg cholesterol; 10 mg sodium

Plant-based!

Breakfast MUSE-li

For a quick breakfast, you'll find our handy MUSE-li Mix to be a great alternative to granola, which often has a lot of extra (and unnecessary) added sugar. *Makes 1 serving*

> 1 cup MUSE-li Mix (page 204)
> ¼ apple, peeled, cored, and coarsely grated
> ¼ cup almond milk
> Sliced bananas (optional)
> Raspberries (optional)
> Chia seeds (optional)

In a small bowl, combine the MUSE-li Mix, apple, and almond milk. Top with bananas, raspberries, and chia seeds, if desired.

Per serving: 455 calories; 20 g fat (2 g saturated fat); 68 g carbohydrates; 13 g fiber; 11 g protein; 0 mg cholesterol; 45 mg sodium

Swapping out ¼ cup dairy milk, you save about:
❀ *¼ mile of driving* ❀ *¾ square foot of land*
❀ *9 gallons of water*

10 Green Eater Meter Score

Scrambled Tofu

Tofu takes the place of eggs in this tasty scramble, which pairs well with warm naan bread or tortillas. Consider making a batch of black beans (see page 224) alongside the tofu for an easy-to-assemble, on-the-go breakfast burrito. Because tofu should be pressed to remove excess moisture before cooking, be sure to start the night before if you have a busy morning. *Makes 4 servings*

> 1 (16-ounce) package extra-firm tofu, drained
> 2 tablespoons olive oil
> ½ teaspoon salt

¼ teaspoon ground turmeric

½ small red onion, finely chopped

1 garlic clove, minced

½ teaspoon ground cumin

¼ teaspoon chili powder

½ cup baby spinach, chopped

1 Roma (plum) tomato, chopped

1 tablespoon chopped fresh cilantro

1 teaspoon fresh lemon juice

1. Wrap the tofu in a clean dish towel and place it on a dinner plate. Set another dinner plate on top of the tofu and place a heavy can on top. Refrigerate for at least 1 hour or up to overnight to press out excess liquid. When ready to use, unwrap the tofu and carefully crumble it into large chunks.

2. In a medium skillet, heat 1 tablespoon of the oil over medium-high heat. Add the salt and turmeric, and stir until thoroughly combined and the oil is golden. Add the tofu and cook, stirring occasionally, until the tofu is lightly browned, 3 to 4 minutes.

3. Transfer the tofu to a plate and set aside.

4. In the same pan, heat the remaining 1 tablespoon oil over medium-high heat. Add the onion, garlic, cumin, and chili powder. Cook until the onion begins to soften, 2 to 3 minutes. Reduce the heat to medium and add the spinach. Cook until the spinach wilts, about 2 minutes.

5. Turn off the heat. Return the tofu to the pan. Fold in the tomato, cilantro, and lemon juice and serve immediately.

Per serving: 180 calories; 13 g fat (2 g saturated fat); 6 g carbohydrates; 2 g fiber; 11 g protein; 0 mg cholesterol; 310 mg sodium

Swapping out 6 eggs, you save about: ✿ *2 miles of driving* ✿ *11 square feet of land* ✿ *173 gallons of water*

Oatmeal with Roasted Peaches

These peaches are so delicious and easy to prepare. They also make a great topping for our plant-based pancakes (see page 208), or serve them with a bowl of plant-based yogurt and your favorite granola. *Makes 2 servings*

FOR THE PEACHES

> 1 tablespoon vegan buttery spread (such as Earth Balance)
> 1 tablespoon brown sugar
> ½ teaspoon ground cinnamon
> 2 peaches, split in half, pit removed
> ¼ cup walnuts, chopped

FOR THE OATMEAL

> 1 cup quick-cooking rolled oats
> 2 cups vanilla almond (or other plant-based) milk

TO MAKE THE PEACHES:

1. Preheat the oven to 350°F. Line a rimmed baking sheet with parchment paper.
2. In a small microwave-safe bowl, microwave the buttery spread on high until just melted, 20 seconds. Add the brown sugar and cinnamon, and stir to combine.
3. Place the peaches on one half of the baking sheet and drizzle the butter mixture over them. Use your hands to toss them gently and ensure they are evenly coated. Arrange the peaches cut side down on one side of the baking sheet and scatter the walnuts on the other side. Bake until the peaches are soft and golden and the walnuts are fragrant and toasted, 10 to 12 minutes. Let the peaches rest for a few minutes, then coarsely chop and set aside.

TO MAKE THE OATMEAL:

1. Meanwhile, in a small saucepan, combine the oats and almond milk. Cook over medium heat, stirring frequently, until the oatmeal has thickened, 5 to 8 minutes.

2. Divide the warm oatmeal between two serving bowls. Top evenly with the roasted peaches and walnuts.

> Per serving: 420 calories; 14 g fat (2 g saturated fat); 67 g carbohydrates; 8 g fiber; 10 g protein; 0 mg cholesterol; 160 mg sodium

Swapping out 1 tablespoon butter and 2 cups dairy milk, you save about: ✿ *2 miles of driving* ✿ *6 square feet of land* ✿ *86 gallons of water*

92
Green Eater Meter Score

Pancakes with Mixed Berry Syrup

These fluffy pancakes pack a great fiber boost from their whole grains, and even the homemade syrup! Great for a cozy weekend morning together.

Makes 4 servings

FOR THE BERRY SYRUP

3 cups mixed berries, fresh or frozen

½ teaspoon lemon zest

½ teaspoon fresh lemon juice

¼ cup agave syrup

½ teaspoon vanilla extract

1 tablespoon cornstarch

1 tablespoon cold water

FOR THE PANCAKES

1 cup whole wheat flour

1 tablespoon ground flaxseed

1 tablespoon baking powder

¼ teaspoon salt

¼ cup almond milk

2 tablespoons grapeseed oil, plus more for the pan

2 tablespoons agave syrup

1 teaspoon vanilla extract

TO MAKE THE BERRY SYRUP:

1. In a small pot, combine the berries, lemon zest, lemon juice, agave syrup, and vanilla. Cook over medium heat until the mixture begins to simmer and the berries release their juices, 5 to 10 minutes.

2. In a small bowl, stir together the cornstarch and water until the cornstarch has dissolved. Add the cornstarch mixture to the berry mixture, increase the heat to medium-high, and cook, stirring occasionally, until the berry syrup thickens, 2 to 3 minutes longer. Set aside.

   For a quick weekday syrup, try this kitchen hack: warm fresh or frozen strawberries or raspberries (my kids' favorites), high-quality maple syrup, and a little splash of water in a saucepan.

TO MAKE THE PANCAKES:

1. In a medium bowl, stir together the flour, flaxseed, baking powder, and salt. In a separate bowl, stir together the almond milk, oil, agave syrup, and vanilla. Slowly add the almond milk mixture to the flour mixture and stir until thoroughly combined.

2. Heat a lightly oiled large skillet or griddle over medium-high heat. When the skillet is hot enough that a few drops of water dance on the surface, pour or scoop ¼ cup of the pancake batter into the skillet for each pancake. Cook for 3 to 4 minutes on each side, until golden brown. Transfer the pancakes to a plate, cover loosely with foil, and repeat with the remaining batter. Serve with the berry syrup.

Per serving: 320 calories; 9 g fat (1 g saturated fat); 58 g carbohydrates; 7 g fiber; 5 g protein; 0 mg cholesterol; 530 mg sodium

Swapping out 1 egg and ¼ cup dairy milk, you save about: ✿ *¾ mile of driving* ✿ *2½ square feet of land* ✿ *52 gallons of water*

Rose's French Toast

Paul, a seed-to-table guru, oversees the garden at our ranch outside Santa Barbara and comes to the house to work with our youngest, Rose, once a week. Last fall, they planted wheat together, and after the spring harvest they ground the wheat berries. Then Paul taught Rose how to make bread using a sourdough starter he had on hand. It was so special to see Rose make her first loaf of bread from wheat that she grew and ground herself. She developed this recipe for her daddy after gifting him a special loaf of bread she made for his birthday.

Makes 2 servings

1 cup vanilla soy (or other plant-based) milk
2 tablespoons all-purpose flour
1 tablespoon sugar
1 tablespoon nutritional yeast
1 teaspoon vanilla extract (optional)
½ teaspoon ground cinnamon
2 tablespoons vegan buttery spread (such as Earth Balance)
4 slices day-old whole grain bread, preferably sourdough
¼ cup maple syrup

1. In a large shallow bowl, combine the soy milk, flour, sugar, nutritional yeast, vanilla, if using, and cinnamon.
2. In a large skillet or griddle, melt the buttery spread over medium-high heat. Working in batches, dip a slice of the bread in the milk mixture and place it in the skillet. Cook for 3 to 4 minutes on each side until golden brown. Transfer the French toast to a plate and repeat with the remaining bread. Serve drizzled with the maple syrup.

Per serving: 485 calories; 8 g fat (2 g saturated fat); 93 g carbohydrates; 7 g fiber; 13 g protein; 0 mg cholesterol; 390 mg sodium

Swapping out 1 cup dairy milk, 1 egg, and 2 tablespoons butter, you save about: ✿ *2 miles of driving* ✿ *7 square feet of land* ✿ *121 gallons of water*

130

Green Eater Meter Score

Lemon-Blueberry-Coconut Scones

These scones are just scrumptious, and a huge crowd-pleaser at MUSE during afternoon snack. They call for a flax egg, a mixture of ground flaxseed and water that takes the place of the traditional egg in this recipe. (See the box on page 212 for instructions.)

Makes 12 scones

1 tablespoon ground flaxseed

3 tablespoons warm water

2 cups all-purpose flour, plus more as needed

5 tablespoons vegan buttery spread (such as Earth Balance)

¼ cup sugar

¼ cup unsweetened shredded coconut

2 teaspoons baking powder

½ teaspoon baking soda

¾ cup vanilla almond milk

Zest of 1 lemon

1 tablespoon fresh lemon juice

½ teaspoon vanilla extract

1 cup fresh blueberries

1. Preheat the oven to 400°F. Line a rimmed baking sheet with parchment paper.
2. In a small bowl, stir together the flaxseed and warm water. Set aside and let sit for 10 to 15 minutes, until the mixture thickens.

3. In a food processor, combine the flour, buttery spread, sugar, coconut, baking powder, and baking soda. Pulse until thoroughly combined. Transfer the flour mixture to a large bowl.

4. In a medium bowl, combine the milk, lemon zest, lemon juice, and vanilla. Add the milk mixture and the flax "egg" mixture to the flour mixture. Stir with a spoon until just incorporated. Mix in the blueberries. The dough will be slightly sticky but should pull away from the sides of the bowl; if it seems too sticky, add an extra tablespoon of flour.

5. Transfer the dough to a lightly floured work surface and pat it into a disc about ½ inch thick. Cut the dough into 12 wedges and arrange them 2 inches apart on the baking sheet.

6. Bake the scones until lightly browned, 15 to 18 minutes. Let cool on the baking sheet for 5 minutes before transferring to a wire rack. Serve warm or at room temperature.

Per scone: 125 calories; 3 g fat (1 g saturated fat); 24 g carbohydrates; 3 g protein; 0 mg cholesterol; 150 mg sodium

Swapping out 5 tablespoons butter and ¾ cup dairy milk, you save about: ✿ *1½ miles of driving* ✿ *6 square feet of land* ✿ *133 gallons of water*

141 Green Eater Meter Score

TO MAKE 1 FLAX EGG
(the equivalent of 1 large chicken egg)

In small bowl, stir together 1 tablespoon ground flaxseed and 3 tablespoons warm water; let sit for 10 to 15 minutes, until the mixture thickens. Use as directed in the recipe. Flax eggs can often be used in place of chicken eggs in other baking recipes, too, although it may take some experimenting.

Ben's Apple-Walnut "Mouffins"

Ben is our nanny, and he loves to cook. He is a plant-based maestro when it comes to cooking for kids. When I first went plant-based, I went through all our cookbooks and got rid of the ones that had animal recipes in them. Then Ben said, "Did you get rid of *Joy of Cooking*?" I didn't even think to keep it! So I got another copy, and he took a muffin recipe out of *Joy of Cooking* and just veganized it. He has completely cracked the code on these muffins. He just figured out the ratios and everything.

His delicious muffins (or "mouffins," as the kids call them) are an easy way to make your mornings a little brighter. Consider measuring your ingredients the night before—just plop them together in the morning and they'll be ready before you head out the door. We especially love this apple-walnut combination, but you can substitute about 1 cup chopped dried apricots for the apple and ½ cup pecans for the walnuts, if that's more to your liking. Pears and sliced almonds work nicely too. In all honesty, this recipe is so versatile, you can use just about any combination of fruit and nuts you can imagine!

Makes 12 muffins

2 cups spelt flour
⅓ cup sugar
1 tablespoon baking powder
2 teaspoons ground cinnamon
½ teaspoon salt
1 cup almond milk
⅓ cup maple syrup
⅓ cup vegetable oil
1 teaspoon vanilla extract
1 apple, cored and finely chopped
½ cup chopped walnuts
¼ cup raisins

1. Preheat the oven to 400°F. Brush a 12-cup muffin tin lightly with vegetable oil or line it with cupcake liners.
2. In a large bowl, whisk together the flour, sugar, baking powder, cinnamon, and salt. In a separate medium bowl, combine the almond milk, maple syrup, vegetable oil, and vanilla. Add the wet ingredients to the dry ingredients and stir until just combined (a few lumps are OK—don't overmix, which will make the muffins a bit tough). Stir in the apple, walnuts, and raisins.
3. Divide the batter among the muffin tin (a spring-action, ½-cup ice cream scoop is great for this task). Bake until the tops of the muffins spring back to a light touch, about 15 minutes. Let cool in the pan for a few minutes, then turn out onto a wire rack to finish cooling. Store in an airtight container for up to three days.

Per serving: 220 calories; 9 g fat (.5 g saturated fat); 32 g carbohydrates; 4 g fiber; 4 g protein; 0 mg cholesterol; 240 mg sodium

Swapping out 1 cup dairy milk, you save about:
✿ *1 mile of driving* ✿ *3 square feet of land*
✿ *35 gallons of water*

39 Green Eater Meter Score

Make Your Own Almond Milk

Many store-bought almond milks have additives and stabilizers; some are even rumored to contain as little as 2 percent almonds! If you'd like the purest, freshest, and creamiest version around, try making your own. Look for organic raw almonds (both Walmart and Trader Joe's sell a pound for less than $15), and be sure to keep them in a tightly sealed container in the fridge between batches of milk, as they can spoil quickly.

Place 1 cup raw almonds in a bowl, add water to cover by about 1 inch, and set aside to soak at room temperature overnight or for up to 2 days. Drain and rinse the almonds with fresh water. Transfer the almonds to a high-speed blender (such as a Vitamix) or the work bowl of a food processor fitted with the metal blade. Add 2 cups filtered water. Blend on the highest speed for 2 minutes (if using a food processor, process for 4 minutes). Line a small colander with cheesecloth and set it in a large bowl. Strain the almond milk through the cheesecloth, gathering the cheesecloth with clean hands and pressing tightly to extract as much liquid as possible. Use agave syrup to sweeten the milk to taste, if desired, and refrigerate in a sealed jar for up to 2 days. Makes 2 cups. (Note: It's easy to double or triple this recipe.) You can also save the almond pulp, spread it over a rimmed baking sheet, and dehydrate it in a low oven (120°F –140°F) for 2 to 3 hours to use in baked goods. If your oven doesn't specify temperatures below 200°F, use the "warm" setting and adjust your time accordingly.

LUNCHES

Spinach–Sweet Potato Soup

At MUSE, soup is one of the most popular lunch entrées. A kindergarten student once told Kayla, our chef, "I can't eat this grilled cheese sandwich if there is no soup to dip it in." From that day forward, she made sure that whenever we serve our plant-based grilled cheese sandwiches, we have soup on the side. (Note: This soup contains a lot of coconut fat, which is a saturated fat; please consider it an occasional treat and review the cautions about coconut oil on page 123.)   *Makes 8 servings*

2 tablespoons olive oil
1 yellow onion, chopped

1 garlic clove, minced

2 sweet potatoes, peeled and chopped

2 tablespoons minced fresh ginger

1 teaspoon salt

1 teaspoon ground cumin

1 teaspoon ground turmeric

1 teaspoon ground coriander

3 cups water

2 cups crushed tomatoes

1 (13.5-ounce) can coconut milk

2 teaspoons vegetable base (such as Better Than Bouillon)

1 (10-ounce) package frozen spinach, thawed

¼ cup chopped fresh cilantro

1. In a large pot, heat the oil over medium-high heat. Add the onion, garlic, sweet potatoes, ginger, salt, cumin, turmeric, and coriander. Cook, stirring occasionally, until the potatoes begin to soften, 10 to 15 minutes.

2. Add the water, tomatoes, coconut milk, and vegetable base and stir until thoroughly combined. Reduce the heat to medium and simmer for 20 minutes. Turn off the heat.

3. Drain the spinach in a colander, squeezing out as much liquid as possible, then stir into the soup.

4. Transfer about 2 cups of the soup to a bowl. Use an immersion blender to puree the soup remaining in the pot until smooth, then return the reserved 2 cups soup to the pot and stir to combine. Stir in the cilantro and serve.

Per serving: 195 calories; 14 g fat (10 g saturated fat);
16 g carbohydrates; 4 g fiber; 4 g protein;
0 mg cholesterol; 630 mg sodium

Plant-based!

Saranne's Roasted "Cream" of Tomato Soup

New Zealand chef Saranne James sometimes cooks for us when we are in New Zealand, and she shared her thoughts about this soup, one of her family's favorites: "A plant-based diet is very important to me, not solely for the health of our planet and our bodies, but also because of the spiritual and elemental connection that is so often overlooked regarding our Mother Earth and all that entails. This soup is so hearty and nourishing, and provides an interesting dimension of taste. For me, there's something about this soup that reminds me of the heartland and home. My mom used to cook us tomato soup when we were sick, so this soup is like love in a bowl."

The kids always *beg* for this when Saranne cooks for us.

Makes 6 servings

> 3 pounds Roma (plum) tomatoes, quartered
> 1 yellow onion, chopped
> 2 tablespoons olive oil
> 4 cups almond milk
> Juice of ½ lemon
> 2 tablespoons tomato paste (optional)
> 2 teaspoons salt
> 1½ teaspoons sugar
> Freshly ground black pepper

1. Preheat the oven to 400°F. Line a rimmed baking sheet with parchment paper.
2. Arrange the tomatoes, cut side up, and the onion on the baking sheet. Drizzle with the oil and toss gently with your hands to coat. Roast until the tomatoes are tender, 30 minutes. Let cool for 20 minutes.
3. Carefully transfer the vegetables and any juices from the baking sheet to a blender and blend until smooth. Transfer the vegetable mixture to a large soup pot and heat over medium-high heat. Stir

in the almond milk, lemon juice, tomato paste, if using, salt, and sugar. Season to taste with pepper.

4. Bring the soup to a boil, then reduce the heat to low and simmer for 15 minutes to allow the flavors to combine.

Per serving: 125 calories; 5 g fat (1 g saturated fat); 15 g carbohydrates; 4 g fiber; 3 g protein; 0 mg cholesterol; 710 mg sodium

Swapping out 4 cups dairy milk, you save about:
- ✿ *3½ miles of driving* ✿ *12 square feet of land*
- ✿ *141 gallons of water*

Rio's Marinated Kale Salad

Rio, a MUSE middle school student, is passionate about cooking. He came up with this recipe for a really delicious kale salad. This salad needs a bit of time to rest—anywhere from an hour to overnight—before serving. The sweetness of the fruit balances out the tangy dressing and the slightly bitter kale.   *Makes 4 servings*

FOR THE DRESSING

   2 tablespoons apple cider vinegar

   2 teaspoons agave syrup

   1 teaspoon ground ginger

   ¼ cup olive oil

   1 tablespoon toasted sesame oil

   Zest and juice of ½ lemon

   ½ teaspoon salt

   Freshly ground black pepper

FOR THE SALAD

   6 cups chopped stemmed kale leaves

   ½ cup pine nuts

   1 green apple, cut into thin strips

2 clementines, peeled and segmented, any pits removed
½ cup pomegranate seeds

TO MAKE THE DRESSING:

In a small bowl, whisk together the vinegar, agave syrup, and ginger. While whisking, add the olive and sesame oils in a slow, steady stream and whisk until thoroughly combined. Add the lemon zest, lemon juice, and salt. Season to taste with pepper.

TO MAKE THE SALAD:

1. In a large bowl, toss the kale with just enough dressing to coat (refrigerate the leftover dressing) and massage the leaves for a minute or two. Cover and refrigerate for at least 1 hour or up to overnight.

2. In a small dry skillet, toast the pine nuts over medium-high heat until lightly browned and fragrant, 5 to 10 minutes (keep them moving in the skillet and watch carefully to make sure they don't burn). Transfer to a small plate and let cool.

3. To assemble the salad, add the pine nuts, apple, clementines, and pomegranate seeds to the bowl with the kale. Toss again and add more dressing, if desired. Serve immediately.

Per serving: 235 calories; 19 g fat (2 g saturated fat);
15 g carbohydrates; 3 g fiber; 3 g protein;
0 mg cholesterol; 200 mg sodium

Plant-based!

Melissa's Coodle Cups with Dill-icious Mango Sauce

Melissa Pampanin, assistant to the head of school and school president at MUSE, tried out a plant-based diet in December 2013 as what she thought was just a one-month challenge, to try to heal up some skin issues. Well, one month turned into four-plus years, and she has no plans of ever turning back. Soon after going plant-based, Mel found a more fruit-based approach to the lifestyle and fell in love.

Never heard of a coodle? They're "noodles" made from fresh cucumber! What's most important to know is that these veggie cups are just as fun to make as they are to eat.   *Makes 2 servings*

FOR THE MANGO SAUCE

1 lime

1 cup chopped red bell pepper

2 cups chopped mango

½ cup chopped green onions

¼ cup fresh dill

1 garlic clove

FOR THE COODLE CUPS

3 large cucumbers, peeled and seeded

1 head butter lettuce, leaves separated

¼ cup chopped green onion

2 tablespoons chopped fresh dill

TO MAKE THE MANGO SAUCE:

Slice a small piece from the top and bottom of the lime and sit it flat on your cutting board. Carefully slice away the zest and white pith of the lime until the flesh is exposed. Chop the lime into 4 pieces and place in the work bowl of a food processor fitted with the metal blade. Add the bell pepper, mango, green onions, dill, and garlic. Process until smooth. Set aside.

TO MAKE THE COODLE CUPS:

1. Using a spiral slicer or julienne tool, slice the cucumbers into long "noodles."

2. In a large bowl, combine the coodles and the mango sauce.

3. Divide the coodle mixture among the lettuce leaves and garnish with green onions and dill.

Per serving: 210 calories; 2 g fat (.5 g saturated fat);
47 g carbohydrates; 10 g fiber; 7 g protein;
0 mg cholesterol; 25 mg sodium

Plant-based!

Davien's Superb Krautwich

Davien Littlefield, my dear friend and former manager who lost sixty pounds with a plant-based diet, shared this awesome kitchen hack: "This sandwich is something that I just invented, and every time I serve it to other people, they're blown away by how satisfying it is. Literally holds me for hours." If you crave the tangy/crunchy mix of a Reuben (without the meat and cheese), these quick-to-prepare sandwiches are the ticket. (If you miss cheese, you can always add a slice of Daiya Swiss-style cheese, but try it without first!) Loaded with probiotics, sauerkraut is the unsung hero of the sandwich world.

Makes 2 servings

> 2 teaspoons vegan mayonnaise (such as Vegenaise)
> 4 slices whole grain bread
> 1 cup sauerkraut, drained
> ¼ teaspoon caraway seed (optional)
> 2 teaspoons whole grain mustard
> 2 teaspoons olive oil

1. Spread the mayonnaise over 2 slices of the bread. In a small bowl, combine the sauerkraut and caraway, if using. Divide the sauerkraut between the mayonnaise-covered bread slices. Spread the mustard over the remaining 2 bread slices and set them on top of the sauerkraut, mustard side down.

2. In a large skillet, heat the oil over medium-high heat. Arrange the sandwiches in the pan and cook for 2 to 3 minutes per side, until toasted.

Per serving: 330 calories; 11 g fat (1.5 g saturated fat);
51 g carbohydrates; 8 g fiber; 9 g protein; 0 mg cholesterol; 880 mg sodium

*Swapping out 2 slices dairy cheese and 5 ounces of
beef, you save about:* ✿ *12 miles of driving*
✿ *393 square feet of land* ✿ *644 gallons of water*

1,049
Green Eater Meter Score

DIY Pickled Vegetables

Instead of simply blanching and freezing your surplus vegetables, consider pickling them! As a bonus, you'll enjoy the benefits of gut-healthy probiotics. Start with 1 pound of whatever fresh vegetable you choose, peeled, trimmed, and cut into whatever shapes you like, and two widemouthed pint jars (with lids) that you've carefully washed and dried. Pack the vegetables loosely into the jars, along with about 1 teaspoon whole spices (mustard seed, fennel seed, cloves, and allspice berries are good bets), a bay leaf or sprig of dill, and a few smashed garlic cloves, leaving about ½ inch of headspace at the top. In a small saucepan, combine 1 cup distilled white or apple cider vinegar, 1 cup water, 1 tablespoon kosher salt, and 1 tablespoon sugar (optional; best to use only if you want sweeter results), bring to a boil, and cook, stirring, until the salt has dissolved. Pour the brine into the jars (you might have some brine left over) so that the vegetables are completely covered. Place the lids on the jars, seal them tightly, and let sit until they've cooled to room temperature. Stick them in the refrigerator for at least 48 hours before serving, and use within 2 months.

Fantastic Falafel

These flavorful patties are fun served family style. Letting everyone have the opportunity to assemble their own distinct creation is an excellent way to inspire kids to enjoy their food. If you like your falafel slathered with a savory spread, consider adding either Aaron's Sweet Potato Hummus (page 256) or Aaron's Eggplant Dip (page 252) to your offerings. For a super-simple tahini sauce option, whisk some water, a tablespoon at a time, into ½ cup tahini until it reaches the desired consistency, then season to taste with garlic powder, a squeeze of lemon juice, and salt. (And if you're using canned chickpeas, save the liquid from the can if you want to make Saranne's Meringues, page 273. You won't regret it.)   *Makes 6 servings*

> ¼ cup plus 1 tablespoon olive oil
> 1 onion, chopped
> 4 garlic cloves, minced
> 1 teaspoon ground cumin
> 1 teaspoon chili powder
> ¼ teaspoon ground turmeric
> 4 cups cooked chickpeas, rinsed and drained
> ½ cup whole wheat flour
> ¼ cup chopped fresh parsley
> ¼ cup chopped fresh cilantro
> 1 teaspoon salt
> 6 whole wheat pitas
> 12 butter lettuce leaves
> 1 cup chopped tomatoes
> ¼ cup chopped red onion
> ¼ cup Kalamata olives, pitted and chopped
> 1 cup chopped cucumbers

1. In a large skillet, heat 1 tablespoon of the oil over medium-high heat. Add the onion, garlic, cumin, chili powder, and turmeric. Cook until the onion softens, 4 to 5 minutes. Transfer the onion to the work bowl of a food processor fitted with the metal blade.
2. Add the chickpeas, flour, parsley, cilantro, and salt. Pulse until smooth, stopping occasionally to scrape down the sides of the bowl.

3. With a clean paper towel, wipe out the pan you used to cook the onion. Heat 1 tablespoon of the oil over medium-high heat. Using a tablespoon measure, carefully place heaping scoops of the falafel mixture in the skillet. Do not overcrowd the pan (six at a time is ideal). Cook the falafel until golden brown and crispy, 3 to 4 minutes per side. Transfer the cooked falafel to a baking sheet and cover loosely with foil. Repeat with the remaining falafel mix, adding 1 tablespoon of the remaining oil to the pan before each batch.

4. Serve the falafel family style and let each person build their own sandwich by topping their pita with the falafel, lettuce, tomatoes, red onion, olives, and cucumbers as desired.

Per serving: 480 calories; 17 g fat (2 g saturated fat);
72 g carbohydrates; 14 g fiber; 16 g protein;
0 mg cholesterol; 960 mg sodium

Plant-based!

Basic Black Beans

You may want to keep a batch of these beans tucked away in the fridge; they add a great fiber and flavor boost to just about anything, from breakfast burritos to nachos. In a pinch, fold a few spoonfuls into some leftover brown rice, and you'll have an easy side dish that's ready to warm up in minutes flat.

Makes 4 servings (about 2 cups)

1 tablespoon olive oil
½ red onion, finely chopped
½ red bell pepper, finely chopped
1 garlic clove, minced
1 (15-ounce) can black beans, rinsed and drained
½ teaspoon salt

½ teaspoon ground cumin

¼ teaspoon chili powder

In a medium skillet, heat the oil over medium-high heat. Add the onion, bell pepper, and garlic and cook, stirring occasionally until the vegetables soften, 2 to 3 minutes. Add the beans, salt, cumin, and chili powder and use the back of a spoon to mash some of the beans. Cook, stirring occasionally until heated through, 1 to 2 minutes longer.

Per serving: 140 calories; 4 g fat (1 g saturated fat);
20 g carbohydrates; 8 g fiber; 7 g protein;
0 mg cholesterol; 440 mg sodium

Plant-based!

MUSE-Y Joes

This recipe is the MUSE kitchen's take on sloppy joes. We use Beyond Meat "beefy" crumbles in place of traditional hamburger meat. These MUSE-Y Joes are just as delicious and satisfying as the real thing, but leave a much softer imprint on the environment.

Makes 4 servings

2 tablespoons olive oil

½ yellow onion, finely chopped

1 green bell pepper, seeded and finely chopped

1 teaspoon paprika

1 teaspoon chili powder

1 teaspoon curry powder

1 (10-ounce) package vegan "beefy" crumbles
   (such as Beyond Meat)

¼ cup ketchup

1 tablespoon whole grain mustard

4 whole wheat hamburger buns

1. In a large skillet, heat the oil over medium-high heat. Add the onion, bell pepper, paprika, chili powder, and curry powder. Cook until the onion softens, 3 to 4 minutes.
2. Add the "beefy" crumbles to the pan and cook, stirring occasionally, until the crumbles have thawed, about 2 minutes. Reduce the heat to low, stir in the ketchup and mustard, and cook until the mixture is heated through, 1 to 2 minutes longer.
3. Divide the "beef" mixture among the hamburger buns and serve.

Per serving: 290 calories; 9 g fat (1 g saturated fat); 27 g carbohydrates; 6 g fiber; 21 g protein; 0 mg cholesterol; 750 mg sodium

Swapping out 10 ounces of beef, you save about:
❁ *20 miles of driving* ❁ *775 square feet of land*
❁ *1,067 gallons of water*

1,159 Green Eater Meter Score

Ree Ree's Raw Vegan Taco Nut "Meat"

My sister Rebecca ("Ree Ree" to family) and I have been on the plant-based journey together for many years. This staple has converted many a beef eater to the plant side. The heartiness and heaviness of the nuts, their protein and fat mixed with familiar spices . . . it's unbelievable how much this mixture tastes like taco meat! It's also wonderful folded into a quesadilla with your favorite dairy-free cheese or served as part of a taco bar buffet. If you only have oil-packed sun-dried tomatoes on hand, just add a little less oil in exchange. Make a batch early in the morning and refrigerate; the flavors really set and improve after 6 to 12 hours.   *Makes 4 servings*

½ *cup raw almonds*
½ *cup raw walnuts*
⅓ *cup loosely packed sun-dried tomatoes*
2 tablespoons olive oil

½ teaspoon salt
½ teaspoon chili powder
¼ teaspoon cayenne pepper (optional)

In the work bowl of a food processor fitted with the metal blade, combine the almonds, walnuts, tomatoes, oil, salt, chili powder, and cayenne, if using. Pulse until the nut mixture is broken down to the consistency of cooked hamburger. Transfer the nut mixture to an airtight container and refrigerate until ready to serve.

Per serving: 260 calories; 24 g fat (2 g saturated fat); 8 g carbohydrates; 4 g fiber; 6 g protein; 0 mg cholesterol; 390 mg sodium

Swapping out 10 ounces of beef, you save about:
❀ *18 miles of driving* ❀ *767 square feet of land*
❀ *994 gallons of water*

1,179 Green Eater Meter Score

"Chicken" Fajitas

This hearty, satisfying classic helps convince many a skeptic that this plant-based thing is totally doable. And while you're eating, take a bit of inspiration from my friend Kathy Freston, who says it best in her wonderful book *Veganist*: "It is safe to say whether we are talking about trimming down, living longer and better, reducing animal suffering, helping the global poor, or shrinking our carbon footprint, there are few things you can do that have the broad impact of a plant-based diet." *Makes 6 servings*

2 (9-ounce) packages vegan grilled "chicken" strips
  (such as Beyond Meat)
Juice of 1 lime
1 teaspoon ground cumin
1 teaspoon chili powder

¼ *cup chopped fresh cilantro*
2 *tablespoons olive oil*
½ *red onion, sliced*
1 *red bell pepper, seeded and sliced*
1 *green bell pepper, seeded and sliced*
1 *yellow bell pepper, seeded and sliced*
12 *spelt tortillas (such as Rudi's)*
1½ *cups shredded vegan cheese (such as Follow Your Heart)*
1½ *cups Really Great Guacamole (page 254)*
Hot sauce (optional)

1. In a medium bowl, combine the "chicken," lime juice, cumin, chili powder, and cilantro. Toss to coat evenly. Set aside.
2. In a large skillet, heat 1 tablespoon of the oil over medium-high heat. Add the onion and bell peppers. Cook, stirring frequently, until the vegetables begin to brown, 8 to 10 minutes. Transfer to a platter and cover loosely with foil to keep warm.
3. In the same pan, heat the remaining 1 tablespoon oil over medium heat. Add the seasoned "chicken" and cook until it is warmed through, 6 to 8 minutes. Add the "chicken" to the platter with the bell peppers and onion and keep warm until ready to serve. Serve the fajitas family style with tortillas, cheese, and guacamole so that everyone can assemble their own. Pass the hot sauce to whomever wants some.

Per serving: 580 calories; 19 g fat (5 g saturated fat); 68 g carbohydrates; 10 g fiber; 30 g protein; 0 mg cholesterol; 980 mg sodium

Swapping out 1½ pounds of chicken and 1½ cups dairy cheese, you save about: ❀ *4½ miles of driving* ❀ *44 square feet of land* ❀ *381 gallons of water*

430

Green Eater Meter Score

Curried "Chicken" Salad in Lettuce Cups

Such a light, refreshing, and ultra-satisfying lunch. The kids at MUSE really enjoy these—they call them "lettuce tacos."

Makes 6 servings

   2 (9-ounce) packages vegan grilled "chicken" strips
      (such as Beyond Meat)
   ¼ cup golden raisins
   3 tablespoons finely chopped red onion
   10 fresh basil leaves, chopped
   2 teaspoons fresh lemon juice
   ½ cup vegan mayonnaise (such as Vegenaise)
   1 teaspoon curry powder
   12 butter lettuce leaves
   Cherry tomatoes, for garnish

1. Chop or tear the "chicken" into bite-size pieces and place them in a large bowl. Add the raisins, onion, basil, and lemon juice and stir to combine.
2. In a separate small bowl, combine the mayonnaise and curry powder.
3. Pour the curry sauce over the "chicken" mixture and stir to combine.
4. Divide the "chicken" mixture among the lettuce cups and garnish with cherry tomatoes.

Per serving: 225 calories; 7 g fat (.5 g saturated fat); 13 g carbohydrates; 4 g fiber; 22 g protein; 0 mg cholesterol; 500 mg sodium

Swapping out 1½ pounds of chicken and ½ cup egg-based mayo, you save about: ✿ *2½ miles of driving* ✿ *42 square feet of land* ✿ *297 gallons of water*

342 Green Eater Meter Score

DINNER SIDES AND MAIN DISHES

Suzy's Family Favorite Chili

This is a mild chili that originated in Canada. Over the years we have altered the ingredients to make it fully plant-based. Feel free to add jalapeños, Tabasco, or other spicy favorites.

Makes 10 servings

2 tablespoons olive oil

6 large white onions, diced

3 (10-ounce) packages frozen "beefy" crumbles
  (such as Beyond Meat)

3 (14-ounce) cans diced tomatoes

3 (15-ounce) cans kidney beans, rinsed and drained

1 (42-ounce) container dairy-free creamy tomato soup
  (such as Imagine Foods)

1 teaspoon chili powder

1. Preheat the oven to 350°F.
2. In a large (6-quart) cast-iron or enameled Dutch oven, heat the oil over medium-high heat. Add the onions and cook until softened, 10 to 15 minutes. Add the "beefy" crumbles and cook, stirring occasionally, until the crumbles have thawed, about 3 minutes. Add the tomatoes, beans, soup, and chili powder. Stir well, transfer to the oven, and bake, uncovered, for 1 hour, stirring every 30 minutes, until it cooks down to chili consistency.

Per serving: 340 calories; 4 g fat (1 g saturated fat); 40 g carbohydrates; 11 g fiber; 29 g protein; 0 mg cholesterol; 900 mg sodium

Swapping out 1 pound 14 ounces of beef, you save about: ❀ *60 miles of driving* ❀ *2,324 square feet of land* ❀ *3,202 gallons of water*

5,586
Green Eater Meter Score

(Wow!)

A KITCHEN HACK FOR THE AGES

This chili recipe comes from Jim's mom, but there's another twist that I added that she'd probably kill me for. (Sorry, Mom Cameron!) One Halloween night, many years ago, I was making chili, as is our annual tradition. When it came time to go trick-or-treating, it hadn't cooked down all the way. *Oh, no!* I thought. *What am I going to do?*

I had an idea: I put the chili in a big cast-iron Dutch oven, stuck it in the oven, turned on the convection, set it at about 300°F–and we went out trick-or-treating! And when we came back, the chili was all cooked. I thought, *OK, this is brilliant.* (Note: To be safe, only do this when someone is home! We'd left some non-trick-or-treaters behind.)

Now if I'm making soups, curries, or sauces, I don't have to sit there and stir to make sure it's evenly cooked, because the convection cooks it from all sides. I'm proud of this kitchen hack–it has served me very well ever since! (Another good hack for chili is to make it in a slow cooker, or even a pressure cooker.)

Mom Amis's Creamed Corn

My mom's growing openness to "vay-gan" eating makes my heart burst. Here's what she says about OMD-ing one of her trademark recipes: "A lot of my family are vay-gan and very healthy as a result! Because my creamed corn is always a favorite, I decided to make a vay-gan version, which tastes just like the original." Now she makes both recipes for big events, and I couldn't be more grateful—it's nostalgia on a plate, a taste of home and family in every bite. (Note: This recipe contains a lot of coconut fat, which is saturated; please consider it as an occasional treat and review the cautions about coconut oil on page 123.)   *Makes 6 servings*

> 6 ears corn, shucked
> ¼ cup coconut oil
> ½ cup Pagie Poo's "Cazzewww" Cream (page 257)
> ½ cup unsweetened almond milk (optional)
> Salt and freshly ground black pepper (optional)

1. Stand an ear of corn on its flat end in a wide bowl or on a rimmed baking sheet and cut downward with a sharp knife to remove the kernels from the cob (don't cut too close to the cob), letting them fall into the bowl. Once you've removed all the kernels, scrape the cob with the side of a spoon to extract the "milk" and corn pulp. Repeat with the remaining ears of corn.

2. In a large skillet, melt the coconut oil over medium heat. Add the corn and the corn "milk" and pulp from the bowl. Cook until the corn begins to soften, about 5 minutes. Reduce the heat to low, add the cashew cream, and simmer until the corn is tender, about 5 minutes longer. If the mixture seems too thick, slowly add a little almond milk until you reach a consistency that you like. Season to taste with salt and pepper.

Per serving: 270 calories; 15 g fat (9 g saturated fat); 33 g carbohydrates; 4 g fiber; 6 g protein; 0 mg cholesterol; 56 mg sodium

Swapping out ½ cup dairy cream, ½ cup dairy milk, and 4 tablespoons butter, you save about: ✿ *2 miles of driving* ✿ *10 square feet of land* ✿ *181 gallons of water*

193

Green Eater Meter Score

Five Brilliant Instant Pot Hacks

Multi-use pressure cookers are a true godsend in the kitchen because they not only make using a pressure cooker super easy (and safe), but also have programmable functions that replace the functions of many other popular appliances, including your slow cooker, rice cooker, and yogurt maker. (They're also another nice way to make chili, an alternative to my "A Kitchen Hack for the Ages," page 231.) Google "vegan Instant Pot meals," and you'll find hundreds of plant-based stews, curries, chilies, soups, risottos, and more. You can prep a whole week's worth of dinners on Sunday, store them in glass containers in the fridge or freezer, throw them in the Instant Pot in the morning, and come home to a piping-hot dinner at night. Definitely follow the manufacturer's safety instructions carefully to make sure you've secured everything correctly. Here's a quick rundown of some staple foods you can easily prepare with an Instant Pot. (The following are tested using a 6-quart model):

Applesauce

Peel, core, and chop 4 pounds baking apples (Granny Smith and Honeycrisp are good choices). Put them in the Instant Pot with 1 cup water, 1 teaspoon lemon zest, ½ teaspoon ground cinnamon, and ¼ teaspoon salt. Seal and cook on High pressure for 8 minutes and then let the pressure release slowly. Stir if you like a chunky sauce; run the mixture through a food mill if you prefer smooth applesauce. Makes about 6 cups.

Beans

Rinse 1 pound dried beans under cold water, drain, and put them in the Instant Pot (no need to soak them). Cover with 8 cups water and add 1 tablespoon olive oil, 1 teaspoon salt, and whatever other seasonings you fancy (garlic, onions, and bay leaves are good additions). Seal and cook on High pressure for 20 to 25 minutes for black beans and black-eyed peas; 25 to 30 minutes for great northern beans, navy beans, and pinto beans; or 35 to 40 minutes for cannellini beans and chickpeas. For best results, let the pressure release naturally. Makes about 5 cups.

Rice

Rinse your rice (at least 1 cup) under cold water, drain, and put it in the Instant Pot. Add an equivalent amount of water (extensive recipe testing indicates that a 1:1 rice-to-water ratio is usually ideal because Instant Pots minimize the usual evaporation that occurs in cooking, but you may want to adjust this amount, as well as cooking times, based on your results). Seal and cook on High pressure for 3 minutes for jasmine rice; 6 minutes for basmati rice; or 20 minutes for brown rice. For best results, let the pressure release naturally. Makes about 3 cups cooked white rice or 4 cups cooked brown rice per 1 cup dry.

Plant-Based Yogurt

Vegan yogurt cultures (available online or in health foods stores) vary by brand, so follow manufacturer's instructions, but in general you'll want to combine 1 packet freeze-dried vegan yogurt culture (refrigerate after opening) with 2 quarts of your favorite shelf-stable plant-based milk, at room temperature. (Look for pure milks with only a few ingredients, such as Pacific Foods, WestSoy, or Edensoy unsweetened organic soy milk– which all have just water and organic soybeans as ingredients– because some additives interfere with the yogurt-making process.) Transfer the mixture to two quart-size mason jars and place in the bottom of your Instant Pot (*not* on the wire rack). Seal and cook on the Yogurt setting for 9 to 12 hours (longer cooking times will result in a tangier yogurt). Refrigerate up to 3 days until ready to serve. Makes 8 cups.

Tomatoes

Set the metal rack inside the inner liner of the Instant Pot and add 1 cup water. Arrange fresh tomatoes on the rack (it's OK to stack them, but don't fill the pot with more than is recommended by the manufacturer). Steam on high for 2 minutes, then use the quick-release function to release the pressure. When the tomatoes are cool enough to handle, their skins will slip off easily, at which point you can use them in your favorite recipes, such as Spinach–Sweet Potato Soup (page 215), or Scooter's Okra and Tomatoes (below), or load them into freezer bags for later use.

Scooter's Okra and Tomatoes

This flavor-packed one-pot dish, traditionally prepared with bacon, is a snap to put together and simply perfect served over your favorite rice blend. If fresh okra is in season, by all means, use it. However, because this dish stews slowly, you'll find a frozen bag of okra works just as well. *Makes 6 servings*

¼ cup grapeseed oil

4 celery ribs, thinly sliced

½ large onion, thinly sliced

2 jalapeños, seeded and thinly sliced

4 to 6 garlic cloves, thinly sliced

Salt and freshly ground black pepper

2 large tomatoes, chopped (about 3 cups)

1 (14.5-ounce) can crushed tomatoes

1 cup vegetable broth

2 tablespoons tomato paste

2 tablespoons red wine vinegar

1 teaspoon finely chopped fresh rosemary
1 pound fresh or frozen okra, stemmed and sliced

1. In a large pot or deep-sided skillet with a lid, heat the oil over medium-high heat. Add the celery, onion, jalapeños, and garlic. Cook, stirring occasionally, until the vegetables soften, 5 minutes. Season to taste with salt and pepper.
2. Add the chopped tomatoes, crushed tomatoes, broth, tomato paste, vinegar, and rosemary and stir well to combine. Bring the mixture to a boil, then reduce the heat to low and simmer for 20 minutes to allow the flavors to combine.
3. Add the okra, cover, and simmer for 20 minutes more, until the okra is tender.

Per serving: 160 calories; 10 g fat (8 g saturated fat); 18 g carbohydrates; 5 g fiber; 4 g protein; 0 mg cholesterol; 277 mg sodium

Swapping out 5 slices of bacon, you save about: ✿ *2 miles of driving* ✿ *13 square feet of land* ✿ *166 gallons of water*

181 Green Eater Meter Score

BBQ "Chicken" Sliders with Classic Coleslaw

Here's a recipe to keep on hand when you are serving anyone who might be skeptical about vegan food. One bite, and you're sure to win them over. And by making your own barbecue sauce, you'll bypass a slew of additives and preservatives. *Makes 6 servings*

FOR THE COLESLAW

½ cup vegan mayonnaise (such as Vegenaise)
2 teaspoons whole grain mustard
1 teaspoon apple cider vinegar
1 teaspoon agave syrup
¼ teaspoon salt
1 (14-ounce) package coleslaw mix

FOR THE BBQ "CHICKEN"

    1 tablespoon olive oil

    ½ yellow onion, finely chopped

    1 garlic clove, minced

    ¼ teaspoon red pepper flakes

    1 tablespoon whole grain mustard

    1 tablespoon apple cider vinegar

    2 teaspoons molasses

    ½ teaspoon garlic powder

    ½ teaspoon smoked paprika

    2 (9-ounce) packages vegan grilled "chicken" strips
        (such as Beyond Meat or Gardein), chopped

    6 whole wheat hamburger buns

TO MAKE THE COLESLAW:

In a large bowl, whisk together the mayonnaise, mustard, vinegar, agave syrup, and salt. Add the coleslaw mix and toss until thoroughly combined. Set aside.

TO MAKE THE BBQ "CHICKEN":

1. In a medium saucepan, heat the oil over medium-high heat. Add the onion, garlic, and red pepper flakes. Cook until the onion begins to soften, 3 to 4 minutes. Add the mustard, vinegar, molasses, garlic powder, and paprika and stir until thoroughly combined. Stir in the "chicken" and cook until warmed through, about 4 minutes.

2. Divide the BBQ "chicken" evenly among the hamburger buns and serve topped with equal portions of the coleslaw.

Per serving: 345 calories; 11 g fat (1 g saturated fat); 28 g carbohydrates; 8 g fiber; 25 g protein; 0 mg cholesterol; 820 mg sodium

Swapping out 1½ pounds of chicken and ½ cup egg-based mayo, you save about: ✿ *2½ miles of driving* ✿ *42 square feet of land* ✿ *297 gallons of water*

342 Green Eater Meter Score

Food Forest Organics Burgers

At Food Forest Organics, purveyor of Cameron Family Farms products, "Making the World Better for You and Your Family, One Bite at Time," in Greytown, New Zealand, we serve a lot of delicious plant-based meals. After cooking over twelve thousand meals and talking to customers, Chef Gayle has developed over twenty-five different basic meal options that are popular with meat eaters and plant-powered people alike. "These are nutritional and nourishing basic alternatives to meat and dairy, serving as platforms or bases which are able to be improvised easily, thus suiting family needs, enthusiastic cooks, and connoisseurs," says Gayle. "I am thankful to be involved with plant-based food, sharing the experience of nourishing with nature's abundance helps to inspire people to care for themselves, others, and the gardens around them."

These burgers are made with FFO's standard "Not Meat" Mix, a good base of beans and grains that can be spiced or flavored in many different ways. For example, add 2 teaspoons Cajun seasoning, a splash of hot sauce, and a dash of cayenne if you like a little extra kick in your burgers; alternatively, 1 teaspoon each of cumin, garlic powder, and smoked paprika is a good option if you prefer a Southwestern twist. Hearty and fiber-rich, these burgers are a great way to use up leftover rice and lentils. They're also gluten-free.

For best results, make sure your grains and beans are chilled or at room temperature. Reheat leftover burgers in a dry skillet over medium-high heat until warmed through. *Makes 12 servings*

1 teaspoon ground flaxseed

1 tablespoon warm water

2 cups cooked brown rice

1½ cups cooked lentils

1½ cups hulled sunflower seeds

1 (15-ounce) can red kidney beans, rinsed and drained

½ cup rice flour
½ cup olive oil
1 teaspoon salt

1. Preheat the oven to 350°F. Line a rimmed baking sheet with parchment paper.
2. Place the flaxseed in a small bowl and pour over the warm water. Set aside.
3. In the work bowl of a food processor fitted with the metal blade, combine the rice, lentils, sunflower seeds, beans, flour, oil, and salt. Add the flaxseed mixture and pulse until combined but with some bean chunks still visible. Scoop ⅓-cup portions of the burger mixture from the bowl and shape them into patties. Place the patties on the baking sheet. Bake until lightly browned, 25 minutes, flipping halfway through. Serve with your favorite burger toppings.

Per serving: 310 calories; 18 g fat (2 g saturated fat); 30 g carbohydrates; 7 g fiber; 10 g protein; 0 mg cholesterol; 250 mg sodium

Swapping out 2¼ pounds of beef, you save about:
❀ *77 miles of driving* ❀ *2,794 square feet of land*
❀ *3,935 gallons of water*

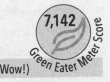

7,142

Green Eater Meter Score

(Wow!)

Open-Faced Peppers

A play on traditional stuffed peppers, these Open-Faced Peppers get a protein boost from beans and quinoa (instead of ground beef), and they remain one of our favorite meals at MUSE. Plus, they're colorful on a plate and easy to complement with just about any side dish. Our chef at MUSE, Kayla, likes to serve these with a side of Jicama Salad (page 241). *Makes 4 servings*

4 large bell peppers, your choice of color
1 tablespoon olive oil
½ red onion, chopped

2 celery ribs, chopped

1 teaspoon ground cumin

½ teaspoon chili powder

½ teaspoon salt

1 cup cooked pinto beans, rinsed and drained

1 cup frozen corn kernels, drained

1 cup cooked quinoa

½ cup chopped fresh cilantro

1 cup shredded vegan cheese (such as Follow Your Heart or Daiya)

1. Preheat the oven to 350°F. Line a baking sheet with parchment paper.

2. Arrange the bell peppers on the baking sheet and bake until they begin to soften, 20 minutes. Set aside to cool.

3. Meanwhile, in a large skillet, heat the oil over medium-high heat. Add the onion, celery, cumin, chili powder, and salt. Cook until the onion begins to soften, 3 to 4 minutes. Add the beans, corn, quinoa, and cilantro. Turn off the heat and stir the bean mixture until thoroughly combined. Set aside.

4. Remove the peppers from the oven and let sit until just cool enough to handle; keep the oven on. Slice the peppers in half lengthwise and carefully remove the stems and seeds. Return the pepper halves to the baking sheet, cut side up. Divide the quinoa filling evenly among them. Top evenly with the cheese, return the peppers to the oven, and bake until the cheese begins to brown, 15 minutes.

Per serving: 320 calories; 13 g fat (1 g saturated fat); 47 g carbohydrates; 10 g fiber; 8 g protein; 0 mg cholesterol; 760 mg sodium

Swapping out 10 ounces of beef and 1 cup dairy cheese, you save about: ❧ *25 miles of driving* ❧ *755 square feet of land* ❧ *1,020 gallons of water*

1,802
Green Eater Meter Score

Jicama Salad

As a side salad, this dish is the perfect crunchy accompaniment to our Open-Faced Peppers (page 239) or any other meal that could use a bright pop of flavor. Jicama, a mild crunchy vegetable similar to a potato but best eaten raw, is a wonderful source of inulin, a soluble fiber that acts as a prebiotic, feeding the beneficial bacteria in your gut.

Makes 4 servings

2 tablespoons olive oil
2 teaspoons fresh lime juice
1 tablespoon chopped fresh cilantro
¼ teaspoon chili powder
1 large jicama, peeled and shredded
1 large carrot, shredded
¼ red onion, thinly sliced
Salt

In a large bowl, whisk together the oil, lime juice, cilantro, and chili powder. Add the jicama, carrot, and onion. Toss to coat. Season to taste with salt.

Per serving: 185 calories; 7 g fat (1 g saturated fat); 29 g carbohydrates; 15 g fiber; 2 g protein; 0 mg cholesterol; 30 mg sodium

Plant-based!

The King's Shepherd's Pie

Rebecca's husband, Jeff King, is the head of MUSE School, and the "OMD" concept was his brainchild. One of Jeff's favorite school lunches is shepherd's pie, so it only seemed fitting to name this plant-based version after him.

Makes 8 servings

6 Yukon Gold potatoes, peeled and quartered
1 cup rice milk

4 tablespoons (½ stick) vegan buttery spread

1 teaspoon garlic powder

3 carrots, halved lengthwise and cut into thinly sliced half-
   moons

3 celery ribs, thinly sliced

½ yellow onion, chopped

1 cup frozen corn

1 cup frozen peas

2 garlic cloves, minced

2 teaspoons dried thyme

2 bay leaves

3 cups cooked brown lentils

2 teaspoons salt

Dash of paprika (optional)

1 tablespoon chopped fresh parsley (optional)

1. Preheat the oven to 375°F. Coat a 13 x 9-inch baking dish with oil.
2. Place the potatoes in a medium pot, add cold water to cover, and bring to a boil. Reduce the heat to medium-low and simmer until the potatoes are fork-tender, 20 minutes.
3. Meanwhile, combine the milk, 2 tablespoons of the buttery spread, and the garlic powder in a small pot and heat over low heat.
4. In a large skillet, melt the remaining 2 tablespoons buttery spread over medium heat. Add the carrots, celery, onion, corn, peas, garlic, thyme, bay leaves, lentils, and 1 teaspoon of the salt. Cook, stirring occasionally, until the vegetables begin to soften, 10 to 15 minutes. Remove and discard the bay leaves.
5. When the potatoes are done cooking, drain them and return them to the pot. Allow the steam to dissipate, 2 to 3 minutes. Add the warm milk mixture and the remaining 1 teaspoon salt. Mash with a potato masher until smooth.

6. Spread the vegetable mixture evenly over the bottom of the baking dish. Top with the mashed potatoes, using a spoon to spread them evenly. Sprinkle the potatoes with the paprika, if desired.

7. Bake until the potatoes begin to brown, 25 minutes. Garnish with parsley, if using, and serve.

Per serving: 295 calories; 2 g fat (.5 g saturated fat); 60 g carbohydrates; 11 g fiber; 12 g protein; 0 mg cholesterol; 880 mg sodium

Swapping out 4 tablespoons butter and 1¼ pounds of beef, you save about: ✿ *19 miles of driving* ✿ *755 square feet of land* ✿ *939 gallons of water*

1,713 Green Eater Meter Score

Cheri and Charlie's Spring Rolls

My brother Charlie loves being plant-based, and this variation on traditional chicken rolls is one of his favorite recipes. Here's what he has to say about it: "I have followed a mostly plant-based diet for about five years now. Now I feel healthier and am more active. I also realize my diet is much better for the environment than eating a bunch of animal products. I'm certainly not a poster child for veganism, but I am honored to be part of the OMD project. One of my all-time favorite meals is this hand roll dinner we served at Jasper's wedding with Suzy and her family. Cheri and I have re-created it at least a dozen times and enjoyed it with our family. It is a super-fun and tasty way to enjoy a meal with people you love. With the right ingredients, it is super healthy as well."

This recipe is so fun to serve family style from many small bowls, letting everyone assemble their rolls the way they want. Once all the ingredients are ready, place a large shallow bowl in the center of the table and stand back (and make sure everyone has clean hands)! *Makes 4 servings*

For the teriyaki sauce

> 2 tablespoons arrowroot powder or cornstarch
>
> 1 cup cold water
>
> ¼ cup reduced-sodium tamari
>
> ¼ cup packed brown sugar
>
> 1 tablespoon agave syrup
>
> 1 garlic clove, minced
>
> ½ teaspoon ground ginger
>
> ⅛ teaspoon garlic powder
>
> 1 tablespoon rice wine (optional)

For the spring rolls

> 2 sweet potatoes, peeled
>
> ½ cup vegetable broth
>
> 2 cups cooked rice noodles or ramen, drained
>
> 1½ cups microgreens
>
> ½ cup spinach
>
> 1 avocado, pitted, peeled, and thinly sliced
>
> 2 bell peppers (your choice of color), seeded and thinly sliced
>
> 1 cup shredded carrots
>
> 16 rice paper wraps
>
> 8 sheets nori seaweed, halved

TO MAKE THE TERIYAKI SAUCE:

1. In a small bowl, stir the arrowroot powder and ¼ cup of the water until thoroughly combined. Set aside.
2. In a small saucepan, combine the remaining ¾ cup water, the tamari, brown sugar, agave syrup, minced garlic, ginger, garlic powder, and rice wine, if using. Cook over medium heat, stirring, until the sugar has dissolved, 2 to 3 minutes (the sauce will appear thin at this point). Slowly pour the arrowroot mixture into the sauce and stir until thoroughly combined. Cook until the sauce reaches the desired thickness; if it becomes too thick, stir in a small amount of water to thin

it. Let the sauce cool to room temperature, then transfer to a small serving bowl.

TO MAKE THE SPRING ROLLS:

1. In medium pot, over medium-high heat, combine the sweet potatoes and vegetable broth. Cover and cook until the potatoes are tender but not mushy, about 25 minutes. Drain the potatoes, slice them into small chunks, and place in a small bowl. Place noodles, microgreens, spinach, avocado, bell peppers, and carrots in similar-size individual bowls.

2. Fill a large shallow bowl with warm water and place it in the center of your serving space.

3. To assemble a roll, soak one sheet of rice paper in the water for 5 to 10 seconds (no longer, or it will get soggy and difficult to work with) and set it on a serving plate. Let sit for about 30 seconds until pliable. Place a nori sheet on top, followed by the desired amount of noodles and other toppings. (Don't make the layers too thick.) Drizzle with teriyaki sauce and carefully fold both ends toward the center, then roll it up burrito style. Enjoy with some extra teriyaki sauce for dipping.

Per serving: 515 calories; 6 g fat (1 g saturated fat); 108 g carbohydrates; 8 g fiber; 8 g protein; 0 mg cholesterol; 680 mg sodium

Swapping out 1 pound of chicken, you save about:

❀ *4½ miles of driving* ❀ *44 square feet of land*

❀ *344 gallons of water*

393 Green Eater Meter Score

Soli and Jasper's Curtido

My son Jasper and his wife, my daughter-in-love, Soli, treat us to food from her native Guatemala whenever they come home to the States. *Curtido* is a spicy cabbage relish that you serve alongside *pupusas* (stuffed and grilled corn tortillas—you can find a plant-based version at https://omdfortheplanet.com/blog/pupusas. Its flavor improves the longer it sits in the refrigerator, so don't hesitate to make it a few days ahead.

Makes 4 servings

½ cup white vinegar

¼ cup water

1 teaspoon salt

1 teaspoon brown sugar

1 teaspoon dried oregano

½ small head cabbage, thinly sliced

2 large carrots, grated

2 jalapeños, seeded and thinly sliced

½ yellow onion, thinly sliced

In a large bowl, stir the vinegar, water, salt, and brown sugar until the sugar has dissolved. Add the oregano, cabbage, carrots, jalapeños, and onion. Toss until thoroughly combined. Cover and refrigerate for at least 4 hours or preferably overnight before serving.

Per serving: 60 calories; 0 g fat (0 g saturated fat); 13 g carbohydrates; 4 g fiber; 2 g protein; 0 mg cholesterol; 625 mg sodium

Plant-based!

Spaghetti Bolognese

Eating plant-based doesn't mean you have to give up on hearty, satisfying meals! If you like a creamier texture, be sure to include the optional cashew cream, which will give the sauce an added boost of richness. Serve with a colorful salad for a dinner that's sure to be a crowd-pleaser.

Makes 6 servings

1 pound spaghetti

1 tablespoon olive oil

2 celery ribs, finely chopped

1 carrot, finely chopped

1 onion, finely chopped

2 garlic cloves, minced

2 teaspoons dried oregano

1 teaspoon dried thyme

1 (10-ounce) package vegan "beefy" crumbles
    (such as Beyond Meat)

1 (28-ounce) can crushed tomatoes

½ teaspoon salt

Pinch of freshly ground black pepper

½ cup Pagie Poo's "Cazzewww" Cream (page 257; optional)

1 tablespoon chopped fresh parsley

1. Cook the spaghetti according to the package directions. Drain and keep warm.

2. Meanwhile, in a medium saucepan, heat the oil over medium-high heat. Add the celery, carrot, onion, garlic, oregano, and thyme. Cook, stirring occasionally, until the vegetables soften, 3 to 4 minutes.

3. Add the "beefy" crumbles, tomatoes, salt, and pepper. Reduce the heat to low and simmer, stirring occasionally, until the crumbles are heated through, 8 to 10 minutes. Stir in the cashew cream, if using.

4. Serve the sauce over the warm spaghetti, garnished with the parsley.

Per serving: 430 calories; 4 g fat (1 g saturated fat); 71 g carbohydrates; 7 g fiber; 23 g protein; 0 mg cholesterol; 697 mg sodium

Swapping out 10 ounces of beef, you save about:
✿ *20 miles of driving* ✿ *775 square feet of land*
✿ *1,067 gallons of water*

1,862
Green Eater Meter Score

Josa's Garlicky Quinoa Salad with Spring Vegetables

Josa has this to share about her yummy recipe: "I've loved to cook for as long as I can remember. When my family went plant-based a number of years ago, I was resistant to the idea; I couldn't imagine altering, or entirely sacrificing, many of the recipes that I loved. Then I spent a lot of time experimenting with my food, began to cook with more vegetables than animal-based proteins, got very comfortable making hummus and cashew cream, and slowly started to realize that these vegan ingredients were just as versatile as anything else I had learned to cook with in the past. Limiting my pantry both allowed and required me to be much more creative in devising meals. As a person who likes to be tested, this challenge, together with the knowledge of the ecological benefit each meal would provide to the world, kept me coming back to plant-based food."

Makes 2 servings

1 small bulb fennel, trimmed, halved, and thinly sliced

1 small sweet onion, finely chopped

2 teaspoons vadouvan curry powder

Salt and freshly ground black pepper

4 tablespoons olive oil

½ cup red quinoa

2 tablespoons almonds

2 large garlic cloves

2 tablespoons red wine vinegar

2 baby bell peppers, cored and sliced into thin rings

½ cup snap peas, sliced crosswise

1. Preheat the oven to 450°F. Line a rimmed baking sheet with parchment paper or foil and set aside.

2. Place the fennel and onion on the prepared baking sheet and sprinkle with the curry powder, a generous pinch of salt, a few

grinds of black pepper, and 1 tablespoon of the oil; toss until thoroughly coated. Arrange the vegetables in an even layer and roast for 21 to 23 minutes until tender.

3. Meanwhile, bring a medium pot of water to a boil. Add the quinoa and cook, uncovered, for 16 to 18 minutes. Turn off the heat, drain thoroughly, and return the quinoa to the pot. Set aside.

4. In a small dry skillet over medium-high heat, toast the almonds, stirring frequently, for 2 to 3 minutes until fragrant. Tip the almonds onto a plate, wipe out the skillet, and set aside. When the almonds are cool enough to handle, coarsely chop them and set aside.

5. Using a garlic grating plate (if you have one), grate or mince one clove of garlic until it resembles a paste. Whisk together the garlic, vinegar, and 1 tablespoon of the oil in a large bowl. Season to taste with salt and black pepper. Add the bell peppers and let sit for at least 10 minutes.

6. Slice the other clove of garlic as thinly as possible (using a mandolin or zester, if you'd like). Using the same skillet used for the almonds, heat 1 tablespoon of the oil over medium-high heat. Add the sliced garlic and cook, stirring frequently, for 20 to 30 seconds until browned (watch closely as it burns quickly). Transfer the garlic chips to a paper towel to absorb any extra oil.

7. To the same skillet, add the remaining 1 tablespoon oil. Cook the snap peas, stirring frequently, for 3 to 5 minutes, or until lightly browned and slightly softened. Season to taste with salt.

8. To the bell pepper mixture, add the roasted vegetables, quinoa, garlic chips, peas, and any oil that remains in the skillet. Toss until thoroughly combined. Taste and adjust the seasonings. Garnish with the chopped almonds.

Per serving: 530 calories; 35 g fat (4.5 g saturated fat);
47 g carbohydrates; 11 g fiber; 11 g protein;
0 mg cholesterol; 650 mg sodium

Plant-based!

Brad and Sandy's Sun-Dried Tomato and Asparagus Lasagna

With a deep passion for engaging community through food, Brad and Sandy Elliott have created comforting and familiar Italian classics for the last twenty-five years in their catering business. Shifting their mind-set to emphasize health and the environment, Brad and Sandy now make their signature meals fully plant-based. This plant-based version of one of their old restaurant's recipes is a favorite on the *Avatar* set (where Brad and Sandy cater daily meals for 150 cast and crew members). Please don't let the number of steps hold you back; there are a lot of parts to assemble, but this dish is so sublime, it will convert even the most skeptical folks in your house!

Makes 10 servings

12 lasagna noodles

1 onion, coarsely chopped

4 garlic cloves

2 tablespoons olive oil

1 (16-ounce) package extra-firm silken tofu, drained

¼ cup plus 2 tablespoons nutritional yeast

Juice of 1 lemon

1½ teaspoons salt

2 (8-ounce) jars sun-dried tomatoes, drained

½ cup packed fresh basil leaves

3 vegan Italian sausage links (such as Field Roast; about
    ½ pound), coarsely chopped

2 bunches asparagus (about 2 pounds), chopped

2 tablespoons water

½ teaspoon freshly ground black pepper

1 (8-ounce) package shredded vegan mozzarella
    (such as Follow Your Heart)

2 tablespoons vegan buttery spread (such as Earth Balance),
    cut into small pieces

1. Preheat the oven to 350°F. Coat a 13 x 9-inch baking dish with oil.
2. Cook the lasagna noodles according to the package directions. Drain and set aside.
3. Meanwhile, in the work bowl of a food processor fitted with the metal blade, combine the onion and garlic and pulse until finely chopped. Transfer about half the onion mixture to a small bowl and set aside.
4. In a large skillet, heat 1 tablespoon of the oil over medium-high heat. Add the remaining onion mixture to the skillet and cook, stirring occasionally, until the onion begins to brown, 5 minutes. Return the onion mixture to the work bowl of the food processor and add the tofu, the 2 tablespoons nutritional yeast, lemon juice, and ½ teaspoon of the salt. Process until smooth, stopping to scrape down the sides of the bowl if necessary. Transfer the tofu mixture to a medium bowl and set aside.
5. Rinse out the work bowl and return it to the food processor. Put the tomatoes, basil, and remaining ¼ cup nutritional yeast in the work bowl and pulse until the tomatoes are finely chopped. Transfer the tomato mixture to a medium bowl and set aside.
6. Without rinsing out the work bowl, add the sausage and pulse until finely chopped.
7. In the same skillet you used for the onion, heat the remaining 1 tablespoon oil over medium-high heat. Add half the remaining raw onion mixture and the sausage. Cook, stirring occasionally, until the sausage is browned and slightly crispy, 5 to 8 minutes. Transfer the sausage mixture to a medium bowl and set aside.
8. In the same skillet, combine the remaining raw onion mixture, the asparagus, water, pepper, and remaining 1 teaspoon salt. Cover and cook over medium-high heat until the asparagus is bright green and tender, 2 to 3 minutes.
9. To assemble the lasagna, spread a small amount of the tomato mixture over the bottom of the baking dish. Arrange 4 lasagna

noodles side by side over the tomato layer and top with thin layers of the following: one-third of the tofu mixture, half the sausage, half the asparagus, one-third of the tomato mixture, and ½ cup of the cheese. Repeat in the same order to form a second layer of each ingredient. Top with the remaining 4 noodles, followed by the remaining tofu mixture, tomato mixture, and cheese. Dot the top of the lasagna with the buttery spread. Cover with foil and bake for 30 minutes. Let stand for 10 minutes, uncovered, before serving.

Per serving: 410 calories; 19 g fat (2 g saturated fat); 46 g carbohydrates; 7 g fiber; 20 g protein; 0 mg cholesterol; 1,040 mg sodium

Swapping out 8 ounces of beef, 8 ounces of dairy mozzarella cheese, 15 ounces of dairy ricotta cheese, 2 tablespoons butter, and 2 eggs, you save about: ❀ *43 miles of driving* ❀ *1,283 square feet of land* ❀ *2,316 gallons of water*

3,642 Green Eater Meter Score

SNACKS, SPREADS, AND DIPS

Aaron's Eggplant Dip

Our chef friend Aaron creates many dishes my family cannot live without. If you have a gas stovetop, charring the skin of the eggplant is a wonderful way to impart a smoky flavor to your finished dip. Another option is to use a gas or charcoal grill to char the eggplant. Serve this dip with crackers or crostini.

Makes 12 servings (about 3 cups)

1 large eggplant (about 1½ pounds)
2 tablespoons olive oil
2 garlic cloves, minced
3 large Roma (plum) tomatoes, peeled, cored, and chopped
1 teaspoon salt

1. Preheat the oven to 500°F. Line a rimmed baking sheet with foil.
2. Using tongs, put the eggplant directly over a gas burner set to its highest setting on the stovetop and cook, turning the eggplant occasionally with the tongs, until the skin is charred, 5 to 10 minutes (trim the leaves beforehand if necessary and watch carefully so they don't burn).
3. Transfer the charred eggplant to the baking sheet. Bake until the eggplant is very soft, 25 minutes. Transfer the eggplant to a large bowl and cover the bowl with a plate or plastic wrap. Let sit until cool enough to handle, about 20 minutes.
4. Meanwhile, in a large skillet, heat the oil over low heat. Add the garlic and cook until lightly browned, 2 to 3 minutes. Add the tomatoes, bring to a simmer, and cook for 20 minutes.
5. Remove the eggplant from the bowl; strain any liquid that has accumulated in the bowl and add it to the skillet with the tomato mixture. Remove and discard the eggplant stem and charred skin and flesh, then scoop all the flesh into a separate clean bowl.
6. Mash with a whisk until the eggplant has broken down into a very coarse puree (some shreds of eggplant flesh are OK). Add the eggplant to the tomato mixture. Add the salt, mix well, and cook, breaking up any remaining chunks of eggplant with the side of a wooden spoon, until the flavors combine, 15 to 20 minutes. Serve warm or at room temperature.

Per serving: 40 calories; 2 g fat (.5 g saturated fat);
5 g carbohydrates; 2 g fiber; 1 g protein;
0 mg cholesterol; 200 mg sodium

Plant-based!

Corn Salsa

Fresh corn in season is one of summer's best gifts—and you'll be richly rewarded if you use it in this recipe. However, if fresh corn is not available and you have to use canned instead, the bright flavors of this salsa are still guaranteed to enhance your meal.

Makes 6 servings (about 1½ cups)

2 ears corn, or 1 (11-ounce) can corn, drained
½ green bell pepper, chopped
¼ red onion, chopped
2 tablespoons chopped fresh cilantro
Juice of 1 lime
1 teaspoon olive oil
¼ teaspoon ground cumin
¼ teaspoon chili powder
¼ teaspoon salt

In a large bowl, stir the corn, bell pepper, onion, cilantro, lime juice, oil, cumin, chili powder, and salt until thoroughly combined. Cover and refrigerate until ready to serve.

Per serving: 60 calories; 1 g fat (0 g saturated fat);
13 g carbohydrates; 1 g fiber; 2 g protein;
0 mg cholesterol; 100 mg sodium

Plant-based!

Really Great Guacamole

Many folks transitioning to plant-based eating find that avocados become their meat-free secret weapon. Rich, creamy, and so satisfying, avocados can add body and staying power to any meal. I say, bring on the guac!

This guacamole is the real deal. Enjoy it on a sandwich in place of mayonnaise, alongside Mexican favorites like tacos and fajitas, or simply straight out of the bowl. Its creamy texture and bright flavors are unbeatable.   *Makes 6 servings (about 1½ cups)*

> *2 ripe avocados, pitted and peeled*
> *Juice of 1 lime*
> *¼ red onion, finely chopped*
> *¼ cup chopped fresh cilantro*
> *¼ teaspoon salt*
> *⅛ teaspoon ground cumin*
> *⅛ teaspoon garlic powder*
> *1 Roma (plum) tomato, chopped*

In a bowl, mash the avocados using the back of a fork. Add the lime juice, onion, cilantro, salt, cumin, and garlic powder. Mix well. Fold in the tomatoes gently.

Per serving: 80 calories; 7 g fat (1 g saturated fat);
6 g carbohydrates; 3 g fiber; 1 g protein;
0 mg cholesterol; 100 mg sodium

Plant-based!

Ree Ree's Cheese Spread

Many folks' sticking point when considering plant-based eating is "How will I ever live without cheese?" Well, here's your answer! Rebecca's cheesy-goodness spread is sure to become a staple ingredient in your house. A great nutty alternative to hummus, this spread is excellent on crackers or alongside a selection of fresh and crunchy vegetables, and also makes a fine sandwich spread. Try it on toast, topped with a few slices of garden-fresh tomatoes!

Makes 8 servings (about 1 cup)

> *1 cup raw cashews*
> *½ red bell pepper, seeded and coarsely chopped*
> *⅓ cup hulled sunflower seeds*
> *¼ cup nutritional yeast*

Juice of lemon
½ teaspoon salt
½ teaspoon chili powder
⅛ teaspoon cayenne pepper

1. Place the cashews in a small bowl and add water to cover by 1 inch. Let soak at room temperature for at least 2 hours and up to 8 hours. Drain and rinse the cashews. Transfer to the work bowl of a food processor fitted with the metal blade.
2. Add the bell pepper, sunflower seeds, nutritional yeast, lemon juice, salt, chili powder, and cayenne. Process until the cheese spread is the consistency of smooth peanut butter, stopping to scrape down the sides of the bowl if necessary, about 1 minute. Cover and refrigerate up to 3 days until ready to serve.

Per serving: 130 calories; 10 g fat (1.5 g saturated fat); 8 g carbohydrates; 2 g fiber; 5 g protein; 0 mg cholesterol; 160 mg sodium

Swapping out 2 tablespoons butter and 8 ounces of dairy cream cheese, you save about: ❧ *¼ mile of driving* ❧ *9 square feet of land* ❧ *266 gallons of water*

276
Green Eater Meter Score

Aaron's Sweet Potato Hummus

Warning: This dip is positively addictive and crazy simple to make. If you're working with whole cloves of garlic, don't worry about peeling them first. Serve with pretzel chips or some good seedy crackers. Roasting the lemons intensifies their flavor and leaves you with a caramelized pulp that's easy to squeeze out of the skin.   *Makes 8 servings (about 2 cups)*

2 large sweet potatoes, peeled and coarsely chopped
4 garlic cloves
2 lemons, halved
2 tablespoons olive oil

1 teaspoon salt
¼ cup tahini
¼ cup water

1. Preheat the oven to 375°F. Line a rimmed baking sheet with parchment paper.
2. Put the sweet potatoes, garlic, and lemon halves on the baking sheet. Drizzle with the oil and sprinkle with ½ teaspoon of the salt. Toss with your hands until the vegetables and lemons are completely coated. Spread evenly on the baking sheet and bake, shaking the pan every 15 minutes, until the vegetables are browned but not burnt, 45 minutes. Remove from the oven and let cool slightly.
3. When the vegetables are cool enough to handle, transfer the sweet potatoes to the work bowl of a food processor fitted with the metal blade. Peel the garlic (if still in their skins) and add to the food processor. Squeeze the pulp and juice from the lemons into a small bowl, pick out and discard any seeds, and add to the food processor, along with the tahini and the remaining ½ teaspoon salt. Process until thoroughly combined, stopping to scrape down the sides of the bowl if necessary. With the motor running, slowly stream in the water through the feed tube until the hummus is very smooth. Refrigerate in a tightly sealed container for up to 1 week.

Per serving: 110 calories; 7 g fat (1 g saturated fat);
10 g carbohydrates; 2 g fiber; 2 g protein;
0 mg cholesterol; 310 mg sodium

Plant-based!

Pagie Poo's "Cazzewww" Cream

Page (my Pagie Poo) has been living the plant-based life for several years, and has recently recruited her husband, Ken. Together, they're exploring the healing powers of plant-based foods while Ken recovers from kidney cancer. "I love seeing the powerful plant-based movement and the rapid uptake in a place like Oklahoma City," says Page. "There has been such an amazing growth in awareness of plant-based lifestyles, and mounting evidence shows that a plant-based lifestyle is one that can truly prevent and reverse so many diseases. We love the versatility of cashew (or as we call it, 'cazzewww') cream and all the things you can use it in—salad dressings, pasta sauces, and even creamed corn! The possibilities are endless."

Makes 8 servings (about 2 cups)

> *2 cups raw cashews*
> *Juice of ½ lemon*
> *1 garlic clove*
> *1 tablespoon nutritional yeast*
> *½ teaspoon salt*
> *1 cup water*

1. Put the cashews in a large bowl, add water to cover by about 1 inch and set aside to soak at room temperature for 4 hours. Drain thoroughly, rinse with fresh water, and drain again. Transfer to the work bowl of a food processor fitted with the metal blade.

2. Add the lemon juice, garlic, nutritional yeast, and salt and process briefly to combine. With the motor running, slowly stream in the water through the feed tube until the mixture becomes creamy. Process until smooth, stopping to scrape down the sides of the bowl if necessary, about 1 minute. Refrigerate in a tightly sealed container for up to 1 week.

Per serving: 200 calories; 16 g fat (3 g saturated fat); 11 g carbohydrates; 1 g fiber; 7 g protein; 0 mg cholesterol; 150 mg sodium

Swapping out 2 cups dairy cream, you save about:
❀ *1½ miles of driving* ❀ *10 square feet of land*
❀ *185 gallons of water*

197 Green Eater Meter Score

Jasper's Peanut Sauce

The beauty of this recipe is that you can basically use whatever peanut products you have on hand—roasted peanuts from a jar or your favorite peanut butter will work equally nicely. And the possibilities for using this stuff are virtually endless—slather it over some freshly cooked Chinese noodles, or use it as a spread in a wrap sandwich with seared tofu and fresh cucumbers or as a great dipping sauce for fresh vegetables. You'll be whipping up a second batch before you know it.   *Makes 10 servings (about 2½ cups)*

1½ cups lightly salted roasted peanuts, or 1 cup peanut butter
¼ cup peanut oil
¼ cup seasoned rice vinegar
¼ cup reduced-sodium soy sauce
1 tablespoon grated fresh ginger
1 garlic clove
¾ cup water

In the work bowl of a food processor fitted with the metal blade, combine the peanuts, peanut oil, vinegar, soy sauce, ginger, and garlic. Process for a few seconds to combine. With the motor running, slowly stream in the water through the feed tube and process until smooth, stopping to scrape down the sides of the bowl if necessary. Refrigerate in a tightly sealed container for up to 1 week.

Per serving: 190 calories; 16 g fat (3 g saturated fat);
8 g carbohydrates; 2 g fiber; 6 g protein;
0 mg cholesterol; 470 mg sodium

Plant-based!

Quinn's Pesto

Quinn's pesto is the pride of our family, and in the summer, he just strolls out into the garden to gather the materials for his art. However, the wide availability of hydroponically grown basil means you don't have to wait until your end-of-summer basil patch becomes overgrown to whip up a fresh batch—three store-bought bunches will work nicely. This recipe makes a very thick, rich pesto, perfect for spreading on a sandwich filled with freshly roasted vegetables. If you want to serve it over pasta, you can thin it down with just a splash of olive oil or some of the water you used to cook the pasta.

Makes 8 servings (about 1¼ cups)

> ¾ cup pine nuts
> 4 cups packed fresh basil leaves (from about 3 bunches)
> ½ teaspoon salt
> ¼ cup nutritional yeast
> ¾ cup olive oil

1. In a dry skillet, toast the pine nuts over medium-high heat until golden brown, about 5 minutes. Tip onto a plate and let cool.
2. In the work bowl of a food processor fitted with the metal blade, combine the basil and salt. Process for about 10 seconds. With the motor running, add the nuts and nutritional yeast. Process for 10 seconds more. With the motor running, slowly stream in the oil through the feed tube and process until smooth, stopping to scrape down the sides of the bowl if necessary. Refrigerate in a tightly sealed container for up to 1 week or freeze for up to 3 months.

Per serving: 275 calories; 29 g fat (3 g saturated fat); 3 g carbohydrates; 1 g fiber; 3 g protein; 0 mg cholesterol; 150 mg sodium

Swapping out ½ cup dairy cheese, you save about:
✿ *¼ mile of driving* ✿ *7 square feet of land*
✿ *148 gallons of water*

158
Green Eater Meter Score

Mom Cameron's Chili Sauce

J im's mom has been making this chili sauce for decades, and the family has now adopted it as our family tradition whenever we have a bumper crop of fresh tomatoes on hand. The flavor is reminiscent of a tomato chutney, which makes it the perfect accompaniment for dozens of dishes, including veggie burgers and hot dogs.

Makes 7 pints (96 servings)

¼ cup pickling spice (like McCormick, Frontier Co-op, or
   Simply Organic)

10 pounds tomatoes

6 onions, chopped

3 green bell peppers, seeded and chopped

3 red bell peppers, seeded and chopped

1 celery head (no leaves), chopped

2 cups apple cider vinegar

1½ cups packed brown sugar

3 tablespoons salt

1. Wrap the pickling spice in a small piece of cheesecloth and tie the bundle shut with kitchen twine. Set aside.

2. Bring a large pot of water to a boil. Fill a large bowl with ice and water. Score the bottom of each tomato with a small X. Working in batches of 6 tomatoes at a time, place them individually on a slotted spoon and carefully lower them into the boiling water. Blanch for 30 seconds to 1 minute. Use the slotted spoon to transfer the tomatoes to the ice bath and let cool. When cool enough to handle, slip off and discard the tomato skins, then core and coarsely chop them, placing them in a large bowl. Repeat to blanch all the tomatoes.

3. In a large heavy-bottomed pot, combine the tomatoes, onions, bell peppers, celery, vinegar, sugar, salt, and the pickling spice bundle. Cook over medium heat, stirring occasionally, until

the vegetables soften, 30 minutes. Reduce the heat to low and simmer, stirring occasionally, until the chili sauce reaches the desired thickness, 3 to 5 hours.

4. Remove the chili sauce from the heat and skim off any foam that has accumulated on top. Remove and discard the pickling spice bundle. (If you plan ahead to make extra, check out canning instructions https://omdfortheplanet.com/get-started/resources.)

Note: *If you have a convection fan in your oven, set it to 350°F, place the pot in the oven, and stir every 20 to 30 minutes. This is the same kitchen hack I use for my chili.*

Per serving: 29 calories; 0 g fat (0 g saturated fat);
7 g carbohydrates; 1 g fiber; 1 g protein;
0 mg cholesterol; 80 mg sodium

Plant-based!

A Family Affair

Although Mom Cameron (or Grandma Cameron, to the kids) would probably kill me for this, we cut the sugar in her original recipe in half. Her version called for 3 cups sugar; we used 1½ cups, and it was still crazy sweet.

When we've made it in the past, we've used those "perfect" red tomatoes from the supermarket that look so beautiful in the store but when you get them home, they really don't taste like much. This year, all the ingredients were from our own garden–the celery, forty heirloom tomatoes, the two bell peppers. When Jim opened a jar and tried the sauce, he just kept saying, "It tastes richer and fresher. The color is even different."

This recipe calls for a lot of bodies in the kitchen because you have to chop and dice everything up–you can't just throw in huge chunks of things. You have to cook it in a large pot, and it takes all day long to make. When the kids are around, we all do it together–it's a huge job! This year, it was our little chef maestro Rose, Ben, our friends Cindy and Benita, and me. So fun. Once the sauce was all cooked up, we used this special canning funnel to pour it into little mason jars, then dunked them in a water bath for 20 minutes (check out the canning instructions https://omdfortheplanet.com/get -started/resources to learn how to can your own sauce).

The thing I love most about canning is that moment when you take them out of the bath and the little lids pop–that's when you know the jars are sealed. Such a satisfying sound. We made about a dozen jars, and I have few extras set aside to take to Grandma Cameron.

Pagie Poo's Delicious Salad Dressing

Page's dressing is simply delicious over just about any kind of salad or vegetable slaw! If you don't happen to have any tahini on hand, use 1 tablespoon olive oil and 1 tablespoon toasted sesame oil in its place.

Makes 6 servings (about ¾ cup)

½ cup Pagie Poo's "Cazzewww" Cream (page 257)

2 tablespoons fresh lemon juice

2 tablespoons tahini

1 tablespoon apple cider vinegar

1 teaspoon Dijon mustard

½ teaspoon garlic powder

½ teaspoon celery salt

¼ teaspoon smoked paprika

¼ teaspoon freshly ground black pepper

In a blender, combine the cashew cream, lemon juice, tahini, vinegar, mustard, garlic powder, celery salt, paprika, and pepper. Blend until smooth. Refrigerate in a tightly sealed container for up to 3 days.

Per serving: 210 calories; 16 g fat (3 g saturated fat); 12 g carbohydrates; 2 g fiber; 7 g protein; 0 mg cholesterol; 140 mg sodium

Swapping out ½ cup dairy cream, you save about:
❀ *1 mile of driving* ❀ *6 square feet of land*
❀ *78 gallons of water*

85
Green Eater Meter Score

Aaron's Ranch Dressing

I f you have a kid in the house, you may be wondering how you'll wean them off their ranch dressing addiction when you do OMD. Well, no need! Smart parents can still wield the tangy, irresistible lure of ranch dressing when it's made with a plant-based ricotta and coconut yogurt instead of buttermilk and all the other traditional dairy ingredients. *Makes 8 servings (about 2 cups)*

¾ *cup plant-based ricotta (such as Tofutti Better Than Ricotta Cheese or Kite Hill)*
⅔ *cup unsweetened coconut yogurt*
3 tablespoons vegan mayonnaise (such as Vegenaise)
1 tablespoon finely chopped fresh chives
1 tablespoon fresh lemon juice
1 garlic clove, minced
½ *teaspoon mustard*
½ *teaspoon dried oregano*
½ *teaspoon onion powder*
½ *teaspoon salt*
½ *teaspoon freshly ground black pepper*

In a large bowl, whisk the ricotta, yogurt, mayonnaise, chives, lemon juice, garlic, mustard, oregano, onion powder, salt, and pepper until thoroughly combined. Refrigerate for at least 20 minutes before serving to allow the flavors to combine. Refrigerate in a tightly sealed container for up to 3 days.

Per serving: 65 calories; 2 g fat (2 g saturated fat); 5 g carbohydrates;
0 g fiber; 1 g protein; 4 mg cholesterol; 250 mg sodium

Swapping out ¾ cup dairy ricotta, ⅔ cup dairy yogurt,
and 3 tablespoons egg-based mayo, you save about:

✿ *1¾ miles of driving* ✿ *7 square feet of land*
✿ *103 gallons of water*

112
Green Eater Meter Score

Patsy's Elegant Three-Course OMD

We're very lucky to have a property on the North Island of New Zealand. Before she became the Governor General of New Zealand, our neighbor was Dame Patsy Reddy and her husband, Sir David Gascoigne. We gave them the bag for Christmas 2013, and Patsy and David had coincidentally been hearing a lot about *Forks Over Knives* at the same time. They watched the film and decided to go plant-based the next day, on December 23. Since then, they haven't looked back. "I found the food so enjoyable, and really didn't find it that difficult," she says.

David lost a lot of weight without trying. Diagnosed with prediabetes and a few other age-related health conditions, he was able to stop taking three different medications after three months on a plant-based diet. The doctors were completely astounded by his good blood pressure and cholesterol count. "When you get that kind of encouragement, it's much easier to keep going and to resist the temptations of a juicy steak," says Patsy.

Whenever possible, Patsy and David offer their guests at Government House a plant-based meal option, and these days, about 40 percent of those guests choose it. New Zealanders are becoming much more conscious of the impact of intensive livestock farming, particularly on their waterways, as they and many of their island neighbors are at the mercy of climate change. "There's a clear generational shift going on here," says Patsy. "It's so good to see our younger generation committing to being leaders on this issue."

Patsy's advice for people going plant-based? Don't think all or nothing. "A lot of people who try it worry about how they can't be strict," says Patsy. "I always think of Suzy and say, 'Just do it for one meal a day—it actually works really well.' "

I'm so honored that Patsy contributed this elegant plant-based meal to the OMD collection. While each component is delightful in its own way, you can serve them as a three-course meal for a special occasion.

A SPECIAL EVENT MENU

The recipes I have chosen for Suzy's book are all recipes that we have served at Government House in New Zealand for special dinners, ranging from royal state dinners to celebratory occasions following investiture ceremonies and special commemorations. They all scale well, but we have cut the recipe size down for the soup and main dish to be suitable for six.

We have found these dishes to be universally popular, with the added benefit of being plant-based, so environmentally friendly. They are also healthy—as long as you don't eat too many Pithiviers or lamingtons at once! This can be tricky, as they are very moreish.

Heirloom Tomato Consommé

This consommé is one of my favorite starters for a special or formal dinner. First, it is elegant and tastes delicious. Though it is light and refreshing, a small portion is satisfying and a great appetite whetter. We first served it at a state dinner for the king and queen of the Netherlands. Queen Máxima was so impressed, she asked for the recipe!

For best results, use your favorite heirloom variety of tomato during peak season. However, in a pinch, "stem-on" tomatoes will serve quite nicely.   *Makes 6 servings*

> *8 large tomatoes, cored and coarsely chopped (about 3 pounds)*
> *½ cup packed fresh basil leaves, plus 12 small fresh basil leaves*
>   *for garnish*
> *1 teaspoon minced shallot*
> *¼ teaspoon minced garlic*
> *1 teaspoon freshly ground black pepper*
> *1 teaspoon salt*
> *1 teaspoon sugar*
> *18 heirloom cherry tomatoes, halved*
> *6 tablespoons extra-virgin olive oil*

1. In the work bowl of a food processor fitted with the metal blade, combine the large tomatoes, the ½ cup basil, shallot, garlic, pepper, salt, and sugar. Pulse until the mixture is smooth, stopping to scrape down the sides of the bowl if necessary.

2. Line a large colander with several layers of cheesecloth and set it in a large bowl. Pour the tomato mixture into the colander. When the initial liquid has drained, tie the cheesecloth bundle closed. Slip a long-handled spoon or similar utensil through the bundle and suspend it over the bowl. Refrigerate until completely drained, preferably overnight. Discard the bundle.

3. To serve, divide the cherry tomatoes among six small bowls, drizzle each with 2 tablespoons of the oil, and garnish with 2 small basil leaves. Pour the chilled tomato consommé over the garnish and serve.

Per serving: 135 calories; 14 g fat (2 g saturated fat);
3 g carbohydrates; 1 g fiber; 1 g protein;
0 mg cholesterol; 390 mg sodium

Plant-based!

Parsnip, Hazelnut, and Pear Pithiviers

A Pithiviers (pronounced *pee-tee-vee-YAY*) is a very special way to serve one of the great dishes most Kiwis love—the humble pie! Traditionally made with meat and cheese, this version is plant-based and has a sophistication not normally associated with the average pie. The creamy parsnip sauce is what makes it supremely tasty. For best results, choose small, light-colored parsnips as they tend to be sweetest. Serve with a lightly steamed green vegetable, such as broccolini or green beans.   *Makes 6 servings*

2 cups vegetable broth

2 pounds parsnips, peeled and chopped into ½-inch pieces

¼ cup plus 2 tablespoons olive oil

¼ cup all-purpose flour, plus more for dusting

½ cup hazelnuts

2 shallots, finely chopped

2 pears, peeled, cored, and chopped into ½-inch pieces

⅛ teaspoon dried sage

⅛ teaspoon ground nutmeg

Salt and freshly ground black pepper (optional)

1 (17-ounce) package frozen vegan puff pastry sheets
   (such as Pepperidge Farm), thawed

1 tablespoon vegan buttery spread (such as Earth Balance),
   softened

1. In a 3-quart pot, bring the broth and 1½ cups of the parsnips to a boil over medium-high heat. Reduce the heat to low and simmer for 20 minutes, or until the parsnips are very soft. Let cool for 10 to 15 minutes. Use an immersion blender to puree the mixture until smooth.

2. In a medium skillet, heat the ¼ cup oil over medium-low heat. Add the flour and cook, stirring occasionally with a whisk, until the color has deepened a few shades, 3 to 5 minutes.

3. Add the parsnip puree in small increments, whisking continuously, until all the liquid has been added. Slowly bring the mixture to a boil, still whisking continuously, then reduce the heat to low and simmer until the sauce is thick and creamy, about 3 minutes. If the sauce appears to have any lumps, pass it through a fine-mesh sieve to remove them. Transfer the sauce to a bowl and cover directly with parchment paper or waxed paper to prevent a skin from forming. Refrigerate the sauce until completely chilled, at least 2 hours or up to overnight.

4. In a large dry skillet, toast the hazelnuts over medium-high heat, shaking the pan occasionally, until brown and fragrant, about 5 minutes. Wrap the nuts in a clean, dry dish towel and let steam for 1 to 2 minutes. Rub the nuts in the towel to remove loose skins (don't worry about any that don't come off). Coarsely chop the nuts and set aside.

5. In the same skillet, heat the remaining 2 tablespoons oil over medium heat. Add the remaining parsnips and cook, stirring occasionally, until golden brown and tender, 10 to 15 minutes. Add the shallots, pears, and hazelnuts and cook, stirring occasionally, until well combined, about 5 minutes longer. Add the sage and nutmeg. Taste and adjust the seasoning with salt and pepper, if desired. Remove the skillet from the heat and allow the mixture to cool to room temperature. Once cool, stir the cooled parsnip sauce into the vegetable mixture.

6. Preheat the oven to 400°F. Line a rimmed baking sheet with parchment paper.

7. On a lightly floured surface, roll 1 sheet of the puff pastry into a 10-inch square, then trim the edges to make a 10-inch-diameter round. Transfer the pastry round to the prepared baking sheet. Spread the vegetable mixture in the center, leaving a 1-inch border. Roll out the second sheet of pastry and cut out a slightly

larger round for the top. Set the larger round over the parsnip filling. Brush the edges with a little water and press them with a fork to ensure the pastry is tightly sealed. Score the top of the pastry and decorate as desired with scraps of leftover pastry. Coat the top lightly with the buttery spread.

8. Bake the Pithiviers until deep golden brown, 30 to 35 minutes. Let rest for at least 20 minutes before slicing and serving.

Per serving: 640 calories; 39 g fat (11 g saturated fat); 77 g carbohydrates; 12 g fiber; 9 g protein; 0 mg cholesterol; 500 mg sodium

Swapping out 1 pound of chicken, 8 ounces of dairy cheese, and 1 tablespoon butter, you save about:
✿ *6¾ miles of driving* ✿ *44 square feet of land*
✿ *656 gallons of water*

Dark Chocolate Lamington Cakes with Blackberry Sorbet

Here's another Kiwi classic that has been adapted as a plant-based dessert for a special occasion. The cake is light, with a rich chocolate finish, and it is beautifully matched with the tang of blackberry sorbet and a small dollop of whipped coconut cream. This makes a fabulous birthday treat that appeals to all ages.

Superfine sugar is an excellent choice when making sorbets because it dissolves easily in water. If you can't find it in your grocery store, make your own by grinding a few cups of granulated sugar in your food processor for a few minutes. Do not use confectioners' sugar as a replacement. If you don't have an ice cream maker, Julie's Organic makes a delicious sorbet with organic raspberries that works just as well. For best results, make the cake a day before you plan to serve it. *Makes 16 servings*

For the sorbet

> 1 (10-ounce) package frozen blackberries
>
> 1¼ cups water
>
> 1½ cups superfine sugar
>
> 2 tablespoons brown rice syrup
>
> Juice of 1 lemon

For the cake

> 2 cups all-purpose flour
>
> 1 cup unsweetened cocoa powder
>
> 2 teaspoons baking soda
>
> 1 teaspoon baking powder
>
> Pinch of salt
>
> 2 cups unsweetened soy milk
>
> 2 teaspoons raspberry vinegar
>
> 1½ cups granulated sugar
>
> 1⅓ cups vegetable oil
>
> 2 tablespoons vanilla extract

For the icing

> 2 ounces vegan dark chocolate (such as Enjoy Life Foods)
>
> 1 cup confectioners' sugar
>
> ½ cup unsweetened cocoa powder
>
> ⅓ cup unsweetened coconut cream
>
> 2 cups unsweetened shredded coconut

> Whipped Coconut Cream (page 274; optional)
>
> 1 cup fresh blackberries

TO MAKE THE SORBET:

1. In a 3-quart saucepan, combine the blackberries, water, superfine sugar, brown rice syrup, and lemon juice. Bring to a boil over medium-high heat and cook, stirring occasionally, until the berries soften and release their juices, 3 to 5 minutes. Remove from the heat and let cool for 10 minutes. Use an immersion blender to puree the berry mixture directly in the pot. Strain the mixture

through a fine-mesh sieve into a bowl to remove the seeds and any remaining pulp. Cover and refrigerate for 4 hours until chilled.

2. Churn the chilled berry mixture in an ice cream machine according to the manufacturer's instructions. Transfer to a freezer container, cover, and freeze for at least 4 hours or preferably overnight before serving.

TO MAKE THE CAKE:

1. Preheat the oven to 325°F. Grease an 8-inch-square cake pan with vegetable oil and line it with parchment paper cut to fit.

2. Into a large bowl, sift the flour, cocoa powder, baking soda, baking powder, and salt. In a separate medium bowl, whisk together the milk, vinegar, granulated sugar, oil, and vanilla. Pour the wet ingredients into the dry ingredients and stir to combine. Transfer the batter to the pan and bake until the cake bounces back to the touch and a toothpick inserted into the middle comes out clean, 1 hour 10 minutes to 1 hour 15 minutes. Let cool completely, preferably overnight, before slicing into 2-inch squares.

TO MAKE THE ICING:

1. Place the chocolate in a large heatproof bowl. Set the bowl over a saucepan filled with 2 inches of water, being sure the bottom of the bowl does not touch the water. Bring the water to a simmer over medium-low heat. When the chocolate has melted, add the confectioners' sugar, cocoa powder, and coconut cream. Stir until smooth and glossy. Keep warm.

2. Place the shredded coconut on a dinner plate. Working with one at a time, dip each piece of cake into the warm icing to coat all four sides. Set the cake in the coconut. Use your other hand to sprinkle a small amount of coconut on the top and sides of the cake. Carefully transfer to a wire rack and let sit until firm, at least 15 minutes. Serve with the sorbet, whipped coconut cream, if desired, and fresh blackberries.

Per serving: 575 calories; 26 g fat (4 g saturated fat); 96 g carbohydrates;
5 g fiber; 5 g protein; 0 mg cholesterol; 210 mg sodium

*Swapping out 2 cups dairy milk, ⅓ cup dairy cream,
and 2 eggs, you save about:* ✿ *3½ miles of driving*
✿ *16 square feet of land* ✿ *212 gallons of water*

232 Green Eater Meter Score

BAKED GOODS AND DESSERTS

Saranne's Meringues

Saranne uses aquafaba, the liquid from cans of chickpeas, to make one of our favorite desserts! "The meringue recipe is a great example of being innovative rather than using conventional products," says Saranne. "You can use plenty of ingredients within the plant-based world to supplement or use as an alternative to obtain a similar (or better) result than the animal product original—plus, they are so much healthier for the mind, body, spirit, and soul, as well as the planet."

For an extra-special presentation, serve the meringues topped with fresh fruit, Whipped Coconut Cream (page 274), and Mixed Berry Syrup (see page 208). The kids *love* these—and Jim and I do too!

Makes 24 meringues

> 1 (15-ounce) can no salt added chickpeas, undrained, at room
>   temperature
> ½ teaspoon cream of tartar
> ¾ cup sugar
> ½ teaspoon vanilla or almond extract

1. Preheat the oven to 250°F. Line a rimmed baking sheet with parchment paper (drizzle a few drops of vegetable oil underneath the corners of the parchment, if necessary, to help it lie flat).

2. Drain the chickpeas into a colander set over a bowl. Measure out ½ cup of the liquid and pour it into the bowl of a stand mixer fitted with the whisk attachment (reserve the chickpeas and refrigerate them, along with any additional liquid for another use). Add the cream of tartar to the stand mixer bowl and beat on high until stiff peaks form (this may take up to 15 minutes). Slowly add the sugar, a few spoonfuls at a time, and whip until glossy. Add the vanilla and mix until thoroughly combined.

3. Drop the meringue batter in generous spoonfuls onto the baking sheet, about 2 inches apart. Bake until the meringues are dry and firm to the touch, 1 hour 15 minutes. Let cool on the baking sheet. Store in an airtight container at room temperature for up to 3 days.

Per serving: 26 calories; 0 g fat (0 g saturated fat); 6 g carbohydrates; 0 g fiber; 0 g protein; 0 mg cholesterol; 0 mg sodium

Swapping out 2 eggs, you save about: ✿ *1 mile of driving* ✿ *6 square feet of land* ✿ *86 gallons of water*

93

Green Eater Meter Score

Whipped Coconut Cream

Keep a can of coconut cream tucked away in the back of your fridge, and you'll always be ready to whip up a batch of this vegan whipped cream. It's such an easy way to make dessert feel extra delicious and decadent. Just make sure to use coconut *cream* (not coconut milk).

Makes 12 servings

1 (14-ounce) can unsweetened coconut cream
½ cup confectioners' sugar
1 teaspoon vanilla extract

In the bowl of a stand mixer fitted with the whisk attachment, beat the coconut cream for 2 to 3 minutes, until light and fluffy. With the mixer running, gradually add the confectioners' sugar and vanilla and beat until thoroughly incorporated. Refrigerate leftovers and use within 3 days.

Per serving: 175 calories; 7 g fat (6.7 g saturated fat);
28 g carbohydrates; 0 g fiber; 1 g protein;
0 mg cholesterol; 15 mg sodium

Swapping out 14 ounces of dairy cream, you save about:
✿ *1 mile of driving* ✿ *7 square feet of land*
✿ *147 gallons of water*

155 — Green Eater Meter Score

Suzy's Carrot Cake

The kids love carrot cake, and this is our rockin' carrot cake recipe. We veganized this from an existing recipe by using applesauce, oil, and Ener-G Egg Replacer. And we swapped the icing for vegan cream cheese and vegan buttery spread. Just make sure you find the right cream cheese to use, because they're not all great. Experiment until you find your favorite. (We've included our favorites as suggestions.)   *Makes 16 servings*

FOR THE CARROT CAKE

4 "eggs" (egg replacer such as Ener-G Egg Replacer)
¾ cup water
2 cups whole wheat or spelt flour
1 cup sugar
2 teaspoons baking soda
2 teaspoons ground cinnamon
1 teaspoon salt
1½ cups canola oil (or applesauce, for an oil-free cake)
3 cups shredded carrots (about 1 pound)

FOR THE CREAM CHEESE FROSTING

4 ounces (1 stick) vegan buttery spread (such as Earth
*   Balance), at room temperature*

1 (8-ounce) package vegan cream cheese (such as Kite Hill), chilled

1½ teaspoons vanilla extract

2 cups confectioners' sugar

TO MAKE THE CARROT CAKE:

1. Preheat the oven to 350°F. Coat a 13 x 9-inch baking dish with oil and dust with flour; tap out any excess flour.
2. In a small bowl, combine the egg replacers and water and set aside.
3. In a large bowl, combine the flour, sugar, baking soda, cinnamon, and salt; mix well. Add the oil and egg replacer mixture and stir until thoroughly combined. Add the carrots and stir until thoroughly combined (a handheld mixer works well for all-purpose flour, but can make spelt tough). The batter will be quite thick.
4. Pour the batter into the baking dish and spread it evenly. Bake until the cake bounces back to the touch and a toothpick inserted into the middle comes out clean, 30 to 35 minutes.
5. Let the cake cool completely in the baking dish before frosting.

TO MAKE THE CREAM CHEESE FROSTING:

In a large bowl using a handheld mixer, beat the buttery spread and cream cheese on medium speed until creamy, 2 to 3 minutes, stopping to scrape down the sides of the bowl if necessary. Add the vanilla and beat on low speed. Slowly add the confectioners' sugar, ½ cup at a time, beating after each addition until smooth.

Per serving: 450 calories; 30 g fat (4.5 g saturated fat); 43 g carbohydrates; 4 g fiber; 4 g protein; 0 mg cholesterol; 450 mg sodium

Swapping out 4 eggs, 4 ounces of butter, and 8 ounces of dairy cream cheese, you save about: ✿ *8½ miles of driving* ✿ *36 square feet of land* ✿ *696 gallons of water*

741
Green Eater Meter Score

Pagie Poo's Lemon Cheesecake Mousse

These treats are Page's signature dish—beloved by omnivores and plant-based folks alike! Light and oh-so-lemony, these dairy-free, no-bake cheesecakes are just 100% yum. For an easy presentation, use 3-inch silicone tart molds; they're super flexible, which makes it easy to slip the cakes out. Also, because conventional lemons usually have some pesticide residue on their skin, please try to use organic lemons, if possible. *Makes 8 servings*

1 sleeve graham crackers (about 9 full sheets)
6 Medjool dates, pitted and chopped
Juice of 1 lemon, plus more if needed
1 (8-ounce) package vegan cream cheese (such as Kite Hill)
½ cup cashews
1 tablespoon lemon zest
Juice of 1½ lemons (about ⅓ cup)
¼ cup maple syrup
8 fresh raspberries
2 tablespoons confectioners' sugar (optional)

1. In the work bowl of a food processor fitted with the metal blade, combine the graham crackers and dates. Pulse until the crackers are broken down into crumbs and the mixture is thoroughly combined. Add the lemon juice and pulse again. The graham cracker mixture should hold together when gently pinched; if it doesn't, add more lemon juice, 1 teaspoon at a time, until it holds together.

2. Set 8 silicone mini tart molds (about 3 inches in diameter) on a baking sheet. Divide the graham cracker mixture among the molds. Carefully press the mixture into the bottom and up the sides of each mold to form a crust. Set aside.

3. Wipe out the work bowl and return it to the food processor. Put the cream cheese, cashews, lemon zest, lemon juice, and maple

syrup in the work bowl and process until smooth and creamy, stopping to scrape down the sides of the bowl if necessary, 2 to 3 minutes. Divide the cream cheese mixture evenly among the tarts molds. Cover lightly with waxed paper (because the silicone molds are very pliable, keep them on the baking sheet) and refrigerate for at least 4 hours, or preferably overnight, until ready to serve.

4. Just before serving, use a small spatula to carefully remove the tarts from the molds and set them on individual serving plates. Top each tart with a raspberry and a dusting of confectioners' sugar, if desired.

Per serving: 220 calories; 7 g fat (1.5 g saturated fat); 39 g carbohydrates; 2 g fiber; 3 g protein; 0 mg cholesterol; 135 mg sodium

Swapping out 8 ounces of dairy cream cheese, you save about: ✿ *2 miles of driving* ✿ *-1 square foot of land* ✿ *96 gallons of water*

97 Green Eater Meter Score

Pagie Poo's Chocolate Mousse

Rich and velvety and so satisfying, here's proof that you don't have to give up a chocolate addiction when you choose a plant-based lifestyle. Best of all, this luxurious dessert is a snap to put together. Make sure to use silken tofu, and remember that a soft tofu will give you a very light result, whereas extra-firm tofu will produce a dense mousse. But rest assured: both are equally delicious.

Makes 6 servings

1 (16-ounce) package silken tofu, drained
1 (9-ounce) package vegan chocolate morsels
    (such as Enjoy Life Foods)
1 teaspoon vanilla extract
Fresh berries (optional)

1. Wrap the tofu in a clean dish towel or paper towels and place in a colander. Set in the sink to allow excess liquid to drain from the tofu, about 10 minutes.
2. Meanwhile, place the chocolate in a microwave-safe bowl and microwave on high in 20-second increments, stirring between each, until the chocolate is melted and smooth.
3. In the work bowl of a food processor fitted with the metal blade, combine the chocolate, tofu, and vanilla. Process until smooth, stopping to scrape down the sides of the bowl if necessary, about 1 minute. Transfer the mousse to a serving bowl. Cover and refrigerate for at least 2 hours, or until chilled, before serving. Serve with fresh berries, if desired.

Per serving: 235 calories; 19 g fat (10 g saturated fat); 0 g carbohydrates; 6 g fiber; 6 g protein; 0 mg cholesterol; 0 mg sodium

Swapping out 4 eggs and 2 cups dairy cream, you save about: ✿ *5¼ miles of driving* ✿ *31 square feet of land* ✿ *428 gallons of water*

Food Forest Organics Coco-Mint Slice

These festive triple-layered treats, the brainchild of Gayle, the chef at Food Forest Organics, are perfect for gift-giving! Spirulina powder is an antioxidant supplement derived from seaweed that imparts a brilliant green color to this dish. Make sure to use unsalted hulled pumpkin seeds; their green color also adds to the overall effect. Rice syrup has the consistency of honey but is slightly less sweet; if you find it too thick to pour easily, zap it in the microwave for 20 seconds or so.   *Makes 64 pieces*

FOR THE BASE LAYER

½ cup plus 2 tablespoons rice syrup
1½ cups hulled sunflower seeds

½ cup walnuts

½ cup almonds

½ cup plus 2 tablespoons coconut oil, melted

¼ cup cocoa powder

¼ teaspoon kosher salt

FOR THE MIDDLE LAYER

¾ cup hulled unsalted pumpkin seeds

¾ cup hulled sunflower seeds or cashews

¾ cup rice syrup (see page 279)

½ cup coconut oil, melted

1 tablespoon mint extract

2 tablespoons fresh mint leaves (optional)

2 teaspoons spirulina powder

FOR THE TOP LAYER

1¼ cups vegan chocolate morsels (such as Enjoy Life Foods)

2 tablespoons almond milk

TO MAKE THE BASE LAYER:

1. Preheat the oven to 350°F. Coat an 8-inch-square glass baking dish with a thin layer of coconut oil and line it with a piece of heavy-duty foil or parchment paper, leaving a few inches of foil or parchment overhanging opposite sides of the dish. Coat the foil or parchment with a small amount of coconut oil.

2. In the work bowl of a food processor fitted with the metal blade, combine the rice syrup, sunflower seeds, walnuts, almonds, coconut oil, and cocoa powder. Process until the nut mixture has the consistency of fine bread crumbs. Transfer the nut mixture to the prepared baking dish and pat it evenly to form a crust. Use the bottom of a flat measuring cup (coated lightly with oil) to help make the crust as even as possible. Bake for 10 minutes. Sprinkle with the salt. Let cool for 10 to 15 minutes before adding the middle layer.

TO MAKE THE MIDDLE LAYER:

1. In the work bowl of the food processor, combine the pumpkin seeds, sunflower seeds, rice syrup, coconut oil, mint extract, mint leaves, if using, and spirulina. Pulse until the seed mixture is the consistency of creamy peanut butter, 2 to 3 minutes.

2. Spread the seed mixture evenly over the base layer. Use the bottom of the measuring cup (again coated lightly with oil) to help make the layer as even as possible.

TO MAKE THE TOP LAYER:

Place the chocolate in a microwave-safe bowl and microwave on high in 20-second increments, stirring between each, until the chocolate is melted and smooth. Stir in the almond milk. Spread the chocolate mixture over the middle layer. Cover and refrigerate until firm, at least 3 hours, before slicing and serving. Cut into 1-inch squares and serve, or refrigerate in an airtight container for up to 2 weeks.

Per serving: 125 calories; 13 g fat (4 g saturated fat); 11 g carbohydrates; 2 g fiber; 2 g protein; 0 mg cholesterol; 40 mg sodium

Swapping out 2 tablespoons dairy milk, 1 cup dairy cream, and 1 egg, you save about: ✿ *1½ miles of driving* ✿ *5 square feet of land* ✿ *64 gallons of water*

71

Green Eater Meter Score

chapter 8

Your Time to Shine

I was talking to my sister Page recently. We both agreed that almost every single day, we hear somebody saying, "Oh, I've been vegan for four months." Or "I've completely cut out meat."

I don't think it's one of those *don't pay attention to the white car* things, when you think it and then all you see is the white car. No, plant-based eating is really coming into its own.

Think about the fairly innocuous term *organic*. That used to be one of those snooty, judgy words. Unless you were a hippie wearing Birkenstocks with granola stuck in your teeth, people didn't want to hear you say "organic." And then, seemingly all of a sudden, organic was catching on and was no longer a hippie word. Now it was a matter-of-fact, very concrete, very desirable descriptor of high-quality food. A worthy—if not always attainable—goal for all. Are we seeing the same signs with "vegan"? As the benefits of plant-based diets spread and the most reluctant meat eaters are gradually giving it a chance, I think we just might be.

The market trends are clear. Research by Experian/Mintel indicates that the rate of growth of vegetarianism in the United States is strong, rising 3 percent between 2012 and 2015 to nearly 10 percent. Almost four in ten consumers agree that restaurants should offer more meatless alternatives, pointing to a rising consumer demand for vegetarian options.[1] According to *Supermarket News*, more than a third of all grocery store shoppers buy plant-based "meats," and over a quarter say they have cut down on eating meat in the past year.[2] In a 2017 memo to their suppliers, Walmart urged food companies to increase their plant-based options and target their marketing to people looking for plant-based foods. When Walmart, a retailer with over 4,600 stores in America, goes out of its way to encourage companies to offer more of any type of product, it's safe to say that's a growth industry.

I'm gleeful that plant-based eating is finally coming into its own. I'm really hoping that, with requests like Walmart's and with programs like OMD, we are approaching a tipping point for plant-based foods, similar to the moment when some people started to really think about the efficiency of their cars—not only as a financial matter, but also as a question of environmental responsibility.

Nowadays, the environmental impact of driving is not even a controversial fact anymore. Almost everyone seeks out cars with high fuel efficiencies, and most car manufacturers offer electric options. But don't forget, there was a time not that long ago when the only cars available were gas-guzzlers—every single person your parents knew drove an 8-cylinder, exhaust-spewing tank and thought nothing of burning up a gallon of leaded gas to go 10 miles or less.

Or think of the early days of no-smoking sections, when people laughed at the nonsmoking scolds and whiners and thought nothing of continuing to smoke in enclosed spaces. Remember when the no-smoking section was literally *right next to* the smoking section, and you had to hold your breath as you walked through?

At first, we didn't blink. Yet as time went on, our collective umbrage grew stronger. You'd see that last holdout obliviously fouling your air and think, *Really?* Then, seemingly at one collective moment, people started to become attuned to the injustice of that, and we started asking the right question: Why do a small group of smokers have the right to impact the health and quality of life for everyone else? And now look where we are: people are rarely allowed to smoke *near* any public building, let alone inside one.

In the documentary *Merchants of Doubt*, we learned about how a few unethical scientists have been paid to distort and manipulate data in order to sow "seeds of doubt" and controversy about what should be settled scientific opinion. They've done it with smoking, they've done it with sugar, they've done it with pesticides, and they've most definitely done it with climate change.

I'm not going to lie: I hope whole-food, plant-based eating becomes so much the norm that people don't even think of it as vegetarian or vegan or even plant-based—it's just "eating." We know that when people learn what a difference plant-based eating makes for the health of the planet, they do make changes[3]—that's a great reason to keep speaking up, talking to friends, cooking up plant-based meals to share, and telling everyone you meet why you're doing this.

Climate change doesn't know any religion, race, sex, sexual orientation. It doesn't care if we're Republicans or Democrats, Cowboys or Eagles fans. And hopefully, our ability to hear the truth about meat's impact on the planet will not be influenced by our "team" affiliations, either. When we get the whole truth, we find it much easier to change—that is often all we need to get started.

Although I've been passionately involved in sustainability initiatives for years, I didn't get real clarity on my own mission until sitting at that NGO meeting and visualizing the flower diagram. I knew instantly that this would be the way I could help make the world a better place for *ALL* our children to grow up in.

To me, this is so incredibly personal. From the moment we went plant-based, everything shifted in our lives. Everything. The work that we do, and how we approach it. How we decide where we're going to invest or give to charity. How we're going to start a new business. It's all filtered through that lens of a plant-based lifestyle. From the development of MUSE to the creation of Red Carpet Green Dress to the establishment of Plant Power Task Force to the growth of Food Forest Organics and Cameron Family Farms to the recent opening of Verdient Foods, our pulse-processing plant and organic farm incubator in Canada—my every waking moment is spent thinking of ways to encourage the development of organic plant-based markets and farmers, and to spreading the word about OMD—I am a woman on a mission. I know the food system is overwhelmingly complex and we need a multitude of fixes and changes. From how we grow food to how we treat farmworkers, from how we feed school children to how we support small farmers to how Big Ag has influenced our supposed dietary guidelines and procurement for far too long—the list goes on and on. As global activist and scholar Vandana Shiva says, "Where am I complicit in a war against the Earth? Where are my daily actions part of a devastation of the planet and with it, a devastation of lives of people, because the two go hand in hand." Everything I do is connected back to raising awareness about animal agriculture, and how plant-based nutrition could be the silver bullet solution that will save us all. That commitment has become the foundation of my entire life.

Now, could we do more? Yes. Of course. Everyone can. That's why we drive electric cars and buy carbon offsets for all our flights. That's why Jim installed solar panels on his *Avatar* production studio and has plant-based catering on set, so the films would be zero-emissions productions. But when it comes to taking a bath, for example, I can breathe a little easier and take that bath with less guilt. With OMD, I know that I've already saved 1,800 gallons of water that day just by not eating that burger.

I'm the kind of crazy that will chase a green bean down the garbage disposal so it can end up in the compost instead—one more green bean that can go back to the earth. This has become a way of life. Taking the extra step, looking for ways to shrink that footprint, lighten that environmental load. Looking in the recycling bin to make sure the kids are rinsing out their jars and cans. Taking more meetings by phone, Zoom, or Skype rather than flying across the country. Trying to walk the walk whenever I can, in whatever ways I can.

When I stopped eating meat, I started dreaming again. A week or so after we went plant-based, I turned to Jim and said, "I know this sounds crazy, but—do colors look a little brighter to you?" I felt lighter, clearer. More connected to the world. My son Jasper compares that moment of clarity, energy, and strength that comes with eating plant-based with the moment the Grinch's heart grows three sizes and he finds he has "the strength of ten Grinches, plus two."

As I'm wrapping up the writing of this book, I'm over the moon to report that our daughter Josa has started implementing plant-based foods into her diet. The other day she came into the house and said, "You'll be very proud—I've been fully plant-based for seven days." She says she intends to stay "maybe 95 percent" plant-based, which just warms my mommy heart. And do you recall my brother, Dave, who taunted me with the dangling meat on my sister's boat? A few months ago, Dave called me after a trip to the doctor had revealed his blood pressure was getting a little high. I convinced him to do a plant-based cleanse, and sure enough if he didn't call me back three weeks later, excited as hell, to tell me his blood pressure is back in normal range. These days, he's also starting to dip his toe into the plant-based world, and I couldn't be prouder or more grateful.

I love the idea of OMD helping to grow some hearts and minds. May we all dig deep and find that strength for the work ahead—and joy in the journey together.

If your OMD experience has left you with that same feeling, are you ready to take action? What are some things we could all do to encourage a transition to plant-based eating? Here are a few suggestions—perhaps try a couple of these to start off, and see where your journey takes you:

⊕ At school, speak to the leadership about plant-based meals and snacks. If there is no plant-based option yet, start there. If they haven't yet started a program like Meatless Mondays (or OMD!), gently nudge them in that direction. Once they're a bit more comfortable, suggest they create a plant-based "foundational" meal, and that meat be the optional add-on rather than the default. Encourage and reinforce any teacher who is sharing accurate information about climate change, eating plant-based foods, and how kids can make a difference in their world. Volunteer to help with letter campaigns, petitions, or other means of peaceful, nonviolent protest by older students. Feed their activist tendencies—we will need their energy for action soon enough. Print out the PDF of the OMD card from https://omdfortheplanet.com/take-the-pledge and take it to your school.

⊕ In the store, ask the management to stock plant-based options, buy them consistently, and encourage your friends to do so as well. If there's a product you can only get online, ask your local store if they'll consider carrying it.

⊕ With NGOs, be cautious about how you spend your money. When they send you holiday donation letters, feel free to call and ask them about their position on animal agriculture. Ask them to show you where they've shared those views—and if they haven't, why not? Consciously donate to the organizations who are awake to the crisis and trying to play a productive role in reversing it. Greenpeace and Sierra Club, among others, are becoming more vocal about the connection between animal agriculture and climate change and environmental degradation. Check first before donating.

⊕ Write letters to the editor or op-eds in your local paper whenever you see a moment to connect the local environment with animal agriculture. Enduring a drought? Write a letter about water use by cows. Contending with a flood? Write a letter about the rising sea levels and coastal flooding, triggered by greenhouse gas emissions released by animal agriculture. Be a reliable voice for the earth, whenever and wherever you see the chance. Don't worry about having something fresh and novel to say every time; repetition of these messages will help them break through.

🌏 With your family, teach your children well, as they say. Remember that every time you eat plant-based, you cut the carbon footprint and water footprint of your diet in half! Doing the OMD program together is an absolutely wonderful start. But as you begin the transition to a plant-based lifestyle, make sure you talk with your children about *why* you're doing this—help them to see, feel, and understand the connection as early as possible. Get them connected to nature while they're still in their young, lovey, literal tree-hugging days. That bond will not only help them speak out as they get older, it will serve as a refuge and a place of solace during times when others just don't seem to understand how precious that nature truly is.

Jim likes to say, "Change doesn't come from the leadership down. Leadership only changes when the people wake up and demand that change." And the opportunity to make that change starts today, with focused attention on our food, with choosing to nourish ourselves in ways that help us, help our families, help all the people, help the animals, and help the earth.

And remember, it doesn't matter why you go plant-based— whether it's for your health, the environment, or for the animals . . . everyone wins! A win-win-win situation all the way around!

Thank you for doing OMD. And invite a friend!

Your OMD Resource Well

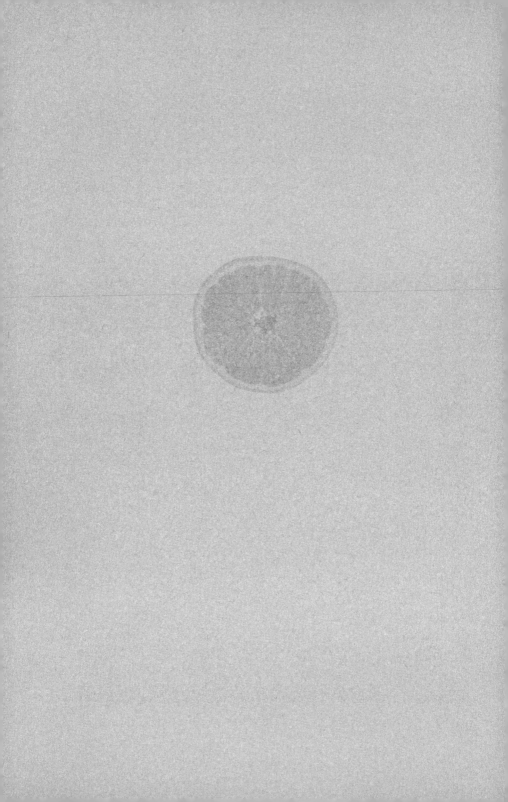

Calculate Your Own
Green Eater Meter Savings

Once you start adding up the Green Eater Meter scores on your meals, you will likely start to see the environmental savings potential in every plant-based dish. Here are the raw calculations for some of the most common animal foods. Find the full environmental savings calculation sheet at https://omdfortheplanet.com/get-started /the-benefits. And then share your own OMD recipes and scores at https://www.facebook.com/OMD4thePlanet/.

If you eliminate . . .	You save this much water . . .	And spare this much land from deforestation . . .	And prevent the release of emissions equal to driving . . .
Beef (2.5 ounces)	285.06 gallons	195.15 square feet	5.36 miles
Butter (1 stick/4 ounces)	173.1 gallons	6.03 square feet	1.23 miles
Butter (1 tablespoon)	21.64 gallons	0.75 square feet	0.15 miles
Chicken (2.5 ounces)	52.94 gallons	6.78 square feet	0.68 miles
Dairy Cheese (1 ounce)	36.98 gallons	1.83 square feet	0.57 miles
Dairy Cheese (1 cup, grated)	147.94 gallons	7.43 square feet	2.26 miles
Dairy Cream (1 cup)	166.09 gallons	12.7 square feet	2.26 miles
Dairy Milk (1 cup)	43.018 gallons	3.98 square feet	1.18 miles
Egg (1)	43.13 gallons	2.91 square feet	0.49 miles

Reusable Food Storage Containers and Utensils

A critical factor in prepping food for busy weeks is having the best food storage containers. To minimize interaction with harmful chemicals leaching out of plastics (as well as to walk the walk in reducing the amount of waste in our world), we try to use glass and stainless steel for everything. (Our favorite brands are Anchor Hocking for glass containers and Zoetica for all manner of zero-waste eating tools.) Here are some essentials that we recommend. Don't feel like you need to go out and buy all of these at once; start with some food containers and go from there:

- Flour sacks
- Glass food containers: Anchor Hocking Bake 'N Take glass dish and lid with optional silicone gasket sleeve (2 cup, 5 cup, 12 cup)
- Glass jars (mason or Ball, many sizes)
- Reusable, compostable food storage bags (such as BioBag)
- Reusable zippered produce bags
- Stainless steel bento boxes
- Stainless steel chopsticks
- Stainless steel coffee mugs
- Stainless steel cups
- Stainless steel straws

The OMD Master Pantry List

These are the products we use on a regular basis; we do try to shake it up for variety and restock as needed. I've suggested brands that are tried and true for our family, and I encourage you to experiment even further. Every day there are new choices available, and every family is unique.

Plant-Based Milks/Creamers

Original Organic Enriched Rice Milk (Dream)

Unsweetened Vanilla Almond Milk (Engine 2)

Unsweetened Original Almond Milk (Engine 2)

Original Hazelnut (Pacific)

Barista Blend Almondmilk (for coffee machine; Califia Farms)

Original Soy Milk (Silk)

Unsweetened Almondmilk (Califia Farms)—cold

Unsweetened Vanilla Almondmilk (Califia Farms)—cold

Original Soy Creamer (Silk)

Vanilla Soy Creamer (Silk)

Plant-Based Cheeses

Miyoko's Creamery

Kite Hill

Daiya

Follow Your Heart

Field Roast

Plant-Based Yogurts

Cashew Yogurt (Forager)

Almond Yogurt (Kite Hill)

Plant-Based Meat Substitutes
Impossible Foods
Beyond Meat
Alfa Foods
Hungry Planet
Field Roast

Nut and Seed Butters
Peanut Butter—Crunchy and Creamy (Santa Cruz)
Almond Butter Raw (Artisana Organics)
Sunflower Seed Butter (Once Again)
Cashew Butter (Artisana Organics)

Packaged Beans and Corn
Garbanzo Beans (Eden Organic or Westbrae Natural)
Traditional Refried Beans (Bearitos)
Black Refried Beans (Amy's)
Black Beans (Westbrae Natural)
Kidney Beans (Westbrae Natural)
Black Eyed Peas (Eden Organic)
Pinto Beans (Eden Organic)
Sweet Corn (Westbrae Natural)
Chili (Amy's)
Organic Chickpeas (One Fig Foods)

Packaged Sauces/Tomatoes
Portabello Mushroom Sauce (Muir Glen)
Italian Herb Sauce (Muir Glen)
Roasted Garlic Sauce (Muir Glen)
Classic Marinara (Muir Glen)
Red Bell Pepper Marinara (Engine 2)

Diced Tomatoes (Radia)

Crushed Tomatoes (Bionaturae)

Packaged Soups

Pumpkin Creamy Soup (Imagine)

Tomato Creamy Soup (Imagine)

Butternut Squash Creamy Soup (Imagine)

Vegetable Broth (Imagine)

Oils/Vinegars/Condiments

Balsamic Vinegar (365 Whole Foods)

Canola Oil—Organic (Spectrum)

Canola Oil Spray (Spectrum)

Dill Pickles—Reduced Sodium (365 Whole Foods)

Grape Seed Organic (Spectrum)

Kalamata Olives, pitted (Mediterranean Organic)

Ketchup, unsweetened (Westbrae Natural)

Old Style Whole Grain Dijon Mustard (Maille)

Olive Oil, organic (365 Whole Foods)

Olive Oil Spray (Pompeian)

Organic Mild Salsa (Enrico's)

Rice Vinegar (Marukan)

Soy Sauce 50% Less Sodium (Tamari)

Soy Sauce Organic (Tamari)

Sweet Relish (Cascadian Farm)

Vegan Caesar (Follow Your Heart)

Vegan Ranch, reduced fat (Follow Your Heart)

Vegenaise Soy-Free (Follow Your Heart)

Yellow Mustard (Westbrae Natural)

Dijon-Style Mustard (Westbrae Natural)

I find beautiful artisanal balsamic vinegars and mustards at farmers' markets too.

Honey/Syrups/Sugars/Jams

Agave Blue Raw and Golden Light Syrups (Madhava)

Brown Rice Syrup (Lundberg)

Clear Stevia (SweetLeaf)

Clover Honey (Topanga Quality Honey)

Creamed Honey (Trader Joe's)

Maple Syrup—Red/Green Grades (Shady Maple Farms)

Strawberry, Red Raspberry, Wild Blueberry,
Black Cherry Jams (St. Dalfour)

Snacks

Apple, Mango, Tangerine Crispy Fruit (Crispy Green)

Blue Chips—no salt (Garden of Eatin')

Brown Rice Snaps (Edward & Sons)

Brown Rice, Wild Rice, Mochi Sweet Rice Cakes (Lundberg)

Corn Snacks (Pop'd Kerns)

Everything Pretzels (Mary's Gone Crackers)

Kids Berry Blast Crispy Rice Bars (Nature's Path)

Kids Strawberry Granola Bars (Nature's Path)

Mango, Blueberry Blast, Mixed Berry Twisted Fruit Snacks
(CLIF Kid)

Popping Kernels (Eden Foods)

Raspberry, Super Orange, Citrus Vitamin Drink Mix
(Emergen-C)

Sea Salt Pretzels (Mary's Gone Crackers)

Seaweed Snack—Sea Salt (GimMe)

Tortilla Chips—no salt (Casa Sanchez)

Vegan Kettle Chips (Earth Balance)

Weetabix (Weetabix)

Zesty Orange Immune Support Supplement (Airborne)

Spices

Cardamom Seed, Ground (Simply Organic)
Cinnamon, Ground (Simply Organic)
Cinnamon Sticks (Frontier)
Vanilla Extract (Simply Organic)

Breads

Spelt Flour Tortillas (Rudi's)
Hamburger Buns (Rudi's)

Assorted Dry Good Staples

Baking Powder (Bob's Red Mill)
Brown Sugar (365 Whole Foods)
Cane Sugar (365 Whole Foods)
French Roast Coffee—Decaf/Regular (Roger's Family Company)
Hemp Hearts (Nutiva)
Organic Ramen Noodles—Asian Vegetable Tofu,
    Garlic Pepper (Koyo)
Powdered Sugar (365 Whole Foods)
Rolled Oats (Bob's Red Mill)
Spaghetti, Penne, Angel Hair Brown Rice Pasta
    (Tinkyada Organic)
Spelt Flour (Arrowhead Mills)

Frozen

Mangoes, Wild Blueberries, Blackberries, Raspberries
    (365 Whole Foods)

Cereals

Unsweetened Blueberry Banana Granola (Sconeage Bakery)
Strawberry Granola (365 Whole Foods)
Raspberry Crunch Granola (Santa Monica Co-Op)

Drinks

Apple Juice (Santa Cruz)

Veggie Juice (R.W. Knudsen)

Tomato Juice—low sodium (R.W. Knudsen)

Sparkling Probiotic Drink (KeVita)

Coconut Water (Costco)

Soft Drinks (Zevia)

Dried Nuts and Fruits

Cacao Nibs (Navitas)

Cacao Powder (Navitas)

Coconut Flakes (organic; any brand)

Dates (Sun Date or 365 Whole Foods)

Almonds (365 Whole Foods)

Brazil Nuts (365 Whole Foods)

Cashews (365 Whole Foods)

Cranberries (365 Whole Foods)

Mango (Costco)

Pecans (365 Whole Foods)

Pine Nuts (Costco)

Pumpkin Seeds (365 Whole Foods)

Slivered Almonds (365 Whole Foods)

Sour Cherries (365 Whole Foods)

Sunflower Seeds (SunRidge Farms)

Walnuts (365 Whole Foods)

Raisins (365 Whole Foods)

Whole Flaxseed (Spectrum)

Personal Care

Nourishing Lavender shampoo, conditioner (Avalon Organics)

Clarifying Lemon shampoo, conditioner (Avalon Organics)

OSEA face and body products

The 14-Day OMD
Transition Plan Shopping List

Here's everything you'll need to prepare your first two weeks of transition recipes. If you're doing this plan to start your OMD program, use this shopping list first, instead of the OMD Master Pantry List. (Note: You'll find a list of all the basic pantry items and staples you'll need for your first two weeks on page 305.)

TRANSITION—WEEK 1

Produce
1 (14-ounce) package coleslaw mix
½ cup baby spinach
1 bunch cilantro
½ cup dried apricots
1 cup chopped dried figs
10 Medjool dates
2 Fuji apples
2 lemons
1 Roma (plum) tomato
1 red bell pepper
1 red onion
1 yellow onion
1 head garlic
1 small hand fresh ginger
Bananas (optional)
Raspberries (optional)

Nondairy and Freezer

1 (16-ounce) package extra-firm tofu
1 (16-ounce) package silken tofu
2 (9-ounce) packages vegan grilled "chicken" strips
2 cups vanilla almond milk

Beans and Grains

1 (15-ounce) can black beans
3 cups rolled oats
1 cup wheat bran
6 whole wheat hamburger buns

Nuts and Seeds

2 cups walnuts
1½ cups roasted peanuts or peanut butter
1 cup raw cashews
⅓ cup hulled sunflower seeds

Additional Items

1 (9-ounce) package vegan chocolate morsels

TRANSITION—WEEK 2

Produce

12 butter lettuce leaves
6 ears corn
3 lemons
1 cup fresh blueberries
1 celery head
1 large tomato
1 cucumber

1 carrot
3 large yellow or white onions
1 small red onion
1 head garlic
1 bunch parsley
1 bunch cilantro

Nondairy and Freezer

5 tablespoons vegan buttery spread
¾ cup vanilla almond milk
½ cup unsweetened almond milk (optional)
1 (10-ounce) package vegan "beefy" crumbles

Beans and Grains

1 pound spaghetti
4 (15-ounce) cans chickpeas
6 whole wheat pitas
2 cups all-purpose flour
½ cup whole wheat flour

Nuts and Seeds

½ cup almonds
½ cup walnuts
2 cups raw cashews
1 tablespoon ground flaxseed

Additional Pantry Items

1 (28-ounce) can crushed tomatoes
⅓ cup sun-dried tomatoes
¼ cup pitted Kalamata olives

YOUR (WELL-STOCKED) OMD PANTRY AND SPICE CABINET

You probably have most of these items on hand already, but here's a list of the extra ingredients you'll need for your first two weeks.

Agave syrup
Apple cider vinegar
Baking powder
Baking soda
Coconut oil
Cream of tartar
Molasses
Nutritional yeast
Olive oil
Peanut oil
Reduced-sodium soy sauce
Seasoned rice vinegar
Sugar
Unsweetened shredded coconut
Vanilla extract
Vegan mayonnaise
Whole grain mustard

Seasonings and Spices

Chili powder
Dried oregano
Dried thyme
Garlic powder
Ground cayenne
Ground cumin
Ground turmeric
Red pepper flakes
Salt
Smoked paprika

The 14-Day All-In Menu Plan Shopping List

Here's what you'll need to make two weeks of delicious vegan meals from our 14-Day All-In Menu Plan. You'll find two lists, broken out by week, as well as a list of the common pantry items and seasonings you'll need for both weeks at the end of this section (most of them you probably already have on hand). If you are only cooking for one or two people, you may find you need fewer ingredients for week 2. If no amount is specified, you only need a very small amount for one of the basic recipes included within the menu plan; feel free to substitute similar foods you may already have for these items as you see fit. (And don't forget to pick up any extra pizza toppings you might like for the recipe on page 158.)

WEEK 1

Produce

- 6 large russet potatoes
- 6 large sweet potatoes
- 7 large bell peppers (2 red, 2 yellow, 2 green, and 1 color of your choice)
- 2 bunches asparagus (about 2 pounds)
- 4 avocados
- 1 large bag chopped fresh kale (at least 6 cups)
- 1 (5-ounce) bag chopped romaine lettuce
- 1 small head broccoli
- 1 cup spinach or stemmed kale leaves
- 1 small bunch basil
- 6 Roma (plum) tomatoes
- 1 bag radishes

2 cucumbers

1 large jicama

2 carrots

2 celery ribs

4 large white onions

2 red onions

1 yellow onion

2 heads garlic

2 bunches cilantro

1 bunch scallions

1 small hand fresh ginger

2 limes

4 lemons

1 bunch bananas

1 mango

1 cup chopped fresh melon

1 pint blueberries

1 pint raspberries

1 pound strawberries

6 Medjool dates

2 apples

¼ cup raisins

Tangerines

Nondairy and Freezer

Vegan butter

2 cups vanilla coconut yogurt

2 (8-ounce) packages vegan cream cheese

2 cups unsweetened almond milk

¼ cup unsweetened nondairy creamer

1 (8-ounce) package tempeh

1 (16-ounce) package extra-firm silken tofu

4 ounces firm tofu

2 (8-ounce) packages shredded vegan cheese (preferably
   cheddar flavor)
1 (8-ounce) package shredded vegan mozzarella
3 vegan Italian sausage links (about ½ pound)
1 package your favorite vegan breakfast sausages
3 (9-ounce) packages vegan grilled "chicken" strips
3 (10-ounce) packages frozen "beefy" crumbles
1 (10-ounce) package frozen spinach
1 small container of your favorite sorbet

Beans and Grains

3 (15-ounce) cans kidney beans
1 (15-ounce) can pinto beans
1 (15-ounce) can vegan refried beans
1 (15-ounce) can chickpeas
12 lasagna noodles
1 sleeve graham crackers (about 9 full sheets)
1 package large flour tortillas (preferably whole grain)
12 spelt tortillas
1 loaf of your favorite whole grain bread
English muffins
1 small baguette
Rolled oats
Quinoa
Brown rice
Whole wheat pitas

Nuts and Seeds

½ cup cashews
½ cup chopped walnuts
Cashew butter
Chia seeds
Ground flaxseed

Peanut butter

Smoked almonds (optional)

Additional Items

2 (8-ounce) jars sun-dried tomatoes

3 (14-ounce) cans diced tomatoes

1 (28-ounce) can crushed tomatoes

1 (32-ounce) package creamy tomato soup

1 (13.5-ounce) can coconut milk

1 (15-ounce) can corn

1 package cornbread mix

1 bag tortilla chips

WEEK 2

Produce

6 ears corn

6 Yukon Gold potatoes

2 large sweet potatoes

5 yellow or white onions

2 bell peppers (1 red, 1 green)

1 pound carrots

1 celery head

1 pound collard greens

6 cups chopped, stemmed kale

1 pound okra (buy frozen if fresh isn't available)

1 small head broccoli

4 large portobello mushrooms

2 (5-ounce) bags arugula

1 cup chopped romaine lettuce

2 large tomatoes

1 pint grape tomatoes

1 cucumber

1 avocado

2 jalapeños

2 heads garlic

3 bunches basil

1 small bunch parsley

1 small bunch cilantro

1 small bunch rosemary

2 lemons

2 peaches

1 pound fresh strawberries

1 bunch bananas

2 Fuji apples

2 green apples

2 clementines

½ cup pomegranate seeds

½ cup dried apricots

1 cup dried figs

10 Medjool dates

Oranges

Grapes

Fresh melon

Nondairy and Freezer

Vegan butter

Vegan cream cheese

1 cup unsweetened rice milk

1 quart unsweetened almond milk

1 quart vanilla almond milk

4 ounces firm tofu

½ package extra-firm tofu

½ cup shredded vegan mozzarella

1 (10-ounce) package vegan "beefy" crumbles

1 cup frozen corn

1 cup frozen peas

3 cups fresh or frozen mixed berries

1 cup frozen pitted cherries

1 small container of your favorite vegan ice cream

1 package of your favorite nondairy ice cream dessert, such as
Tofutti Cuties

Beans and Grains

1 (15-ounce) can red kidney beans

1 (15-ounce) can vegan baked beans

1 (15-ounce) can chickpeas

1 pound brown lentils

1 loaf of your favorite whole grain bread

English muffins

4 whole wheat hamburger buns

1 package large whole wheat tortillas

4 cups rolled oats

1 cup wheat bran

1 cup whole wheat flour

1 cup brown rice

½ cup rice flour

Converted rice

Quinoa

Nuts and Seeds

3 cups raw cashews

2 cups hulled sunflower seeds

2¼ cups walnuts

1¼ cups pine nuts

Chia seeds

Ground flaxseed

Crushed peanuts

Peanut butter

Additional Items
 1 (14.5-ounce) can crushed tomatoes
 1 (15-ounce) can coconut cream
 1 (20-ounce) can brined jackfruit
 ½ cup roasted red pepper strips
 Prepared hummus
 Olives
 Vegan croutons
 Crackers

YOUR (WELL-STOCKED) ALL-IN PANTRY AND SPICE CABINET
You probably have most of these items on hand already, but here's a list of the extra ingredients you'll need for these two weeks:
 Agave syrup
 All-purpose flour
 Apple cider vinegar
 Baking powder
 Balsamic vinegar
 Barbecue sauce
 Brown sugar
 Chocolate sauce
 Coconut oil
 Cornstarch
 Dark chocolate
 Grapeseed oil
 Jelly
 Ketchup
 Maple syrup
 Nutritional yeast
 Olive oil
 Panko bread crumbs
 Pickle relish
 Popcorn

Red wine vinegar
Salsa
Spelt flour
Sriracha sauce
Sugar
Toasted sesame oil
Tomato paste
Vanilla extract
Vegan mayonnaise
Vegetable broth
Vegetable oil
Whole grain or Dijon mustard

Spices and Seasonings

Bay leaves
Black pepper
Cayenne pepper
Chili powder
Chives
Curry powder
Dried thyme
Garlic powder
Garlic salt
Ground allspice
Ground cinnamon
Ground coriander
Ground cumin
Ground turmeric
Onion powder
Paprika
Red pepper flakes
Salt

Converting to Metrics

VOLUME MEASUREMENT CONVERSIONS

Cups	Tablespoons	Teaspoons	Milliliters
		1 tsp	5 ml
1/16 cup	1 tbsp	3 tsp	15 ml
1/8 cup	2 tbsp	6 tsp	30 ml
1/4 cup	4 tbsp	12 tsp	50 ml
1/3 cup	5 1/3 tbsp	16 tsp	75 ml
1/2 cup	8 tbsp	24 tsp	125 ml
2/3 cup	10 2/3 tbsp	32 tsp	150 ml
3/4 cup	12 tbsp	36 tsp	150 ml
1 cup	16 tbsp	48 tsp	250 ml

WEIGHT CONVERSION MEASUREMENTS

US	Metric
1 ounce	28.34 grams (g)
8 ounces	227 g
16 ounces (1 pound)	454 g

COOKING TEMPERATURE CONVERSIONS

Celsius/Centigrade	$F = (C \times 1.8) + 32$
Fahrenheit	$C = (F - 32) \times 0.5555$

Zero degrees Celsius and 100°C are arbitrarily placed at the melting and boiling points of water, while Fahrenheit establishes 0°F as the stabilized temperature when equal amounts of ice, water, and salt are mixed. So, for example, if you are baking at 350°F and want to know that temperature in Celsius, the following calculation will provide it: $C = (350 - 32) \times 0.5555 = 176.66°C$.

Further Reading, Watching, and Learning

If you've been intrigued by the ideas here, I encourage you to keep researching and learning about the damage done by animal agriculture, and the tremendous positive power of plant-based nutrition. I am certain that the more books you read, the more documentaries you watch, and the more you learn about plant-based nutrition, the more inspired and motivated you will become.

BOOKS

GENERAL PLANT-BASED NUTRITION

The China Study Solution: The Simple Way to Lose Weight and Reverse Illness, Using a Whole-Food, Plant-Based Diet by Dr. T. Colin Campbell

Whole: Rethinking the Science of Nutrition by Dr. T. Colin Campbell

Clean Protein: The Revolution That Will Reshape Your Body, Boost Your Energy—and Save Our Planet by Kathy Freston

Quantum Wellness: A Practical Guide to Health and Happiness by Kathy Freston

The Lean: A Revolutionary (and Simple!) 30-Day Plan for Healthy, Lasting Weight Loss by Kathy Freston

Veganist: Lose Weight, Get Healthy, Change the World by Kathy Freston

How Not to Die: Discover the Foods Scientifically Proven to Prevent and Reverse Disease by Dr. Michael Greger

The Healthiest Diet on the Planet: Why the Foods You Love—Pizza, Pancakes, Potatoes, Pasta, and More—Are the Solution to Preventing Disease and Looking and Feeling Your Best by Dr. John McDougall

Meatless: Transform the Way You Eat and Live—One Meal at a Time by Kristie Middleton

The Plant-Based Journey: A Step-by-Step Guide for Transitioning to a Healthy Lifestyle and Achieving Your Ideal Weight by Lani Muelrath

The Spectrum: A Scientifically Proven Program to Feel Better, Live Longer, Lose Weight, and Gain Health by Dr. Dean Ornish

The Plant-Powered Diet: The Lifelong Eating Plan for Achieving Optimal Health, Beginning Today by Sharon Palmer, RD

Healthy at 100: The Scientifically Proven Secrets of the World's Healthiest and Longest-Lived Peoples by John Robbins

The Plantpower Way: Whole Food Plant-Based Recipes and Guidance for The Whole Family by Rich Roll

Finding Ultra: Rejecting Middle Age, Becoming One of the World's Fittest Men, and Discovering Myself by Rich Roll

DIABETES

Dr. Neal Barnard's Program for Reversing Diabetes: The Scientifically Proven System for Reversing Diabetes Without Drugs by Dr. Neal Barnard

FOOD CRAVINGS

Breaking the Food Seduction: The Hidden Reasons Behind Food Cravings—And 7 Steps to End Them Naturally by Dr. Neal Barnard

The Cheese Trap: How Breaking a Surprising Addiction Will Help You Lose Weight, Gain Energy, and Get Healthy by Dr. Neal Barnard

WEIGHT LOSS

Foods That Cause You to Lose Weight: The Negative Calorie Effect by Dr. Neal Barnard

The Engine 2 Cookbook: More than 130 Lip-Smacking, Rib-Sticking, Body-Slimming Recipes to Live Plant-Strong by Rip Esselstyn

The Engine 2 Diet: The Texas Firefighter's 28-Day Save-Your-Life Plan that Lowers Cholesterol and Burns Away the Pounds by Rip Esselstyn

The Engine 2 Seven-Day Rescue Diet: Eat Plants, Lose Weight, Save Your Health by Rip Esselstyn

Plant-Strong: Discover the World's Healthiest Diet—with 150 Engine 2 Recipes by Rip Esselstyn

The Starch Solution: Eat the Foods You Love, Regain Your Health, and Lose the Weight for Good! by Dr. John McDougall

Eat More, Weigh Less: Dr. Dean Ornish's Life Choice Program for Losing Weight Safely While Eating Abundantly by Dr. Dean Ornish

HEART DISEASE

Prevent and Reverse Heart Disease: The Revolutionary, Scientifically Proven, Nutrition-Based Cure by Dr. Caldwell Esselstyn

The McDougall Program for a Healthy Heart: A Life-Saving Approach to Preventing and Treating Heart Disease by Dr. John McDougall

Dr. Dean Ornish's Program for Reversing Heart Disease: The Only System Scientifically Proven to Reverse Heart Disease Without Drugs or Surgery by Dr. Dean Ornish

CLIMATE CHANGE AND ENVIRONMENT

The Sustainability Secret: Rethinking Our Diet to Transform the World by Kip Andersen and Keegen Kuhn

Healthy Eating, Healthy World: Unleashing the Power of Plant-Based Nutrition by J. Morris Hicks

Comfortably Unaware: What We Choose to Eat Is Killing Us and Our Planet by Dr. Richard Oppenlander

Food Choice and Sustainability: Why Buying Local, Eating Less Meat, and Taking Baby Steps Won't Work by Dr. Richard Oppenlander

Voices of the Food Revolution: You Can Heal Your Body and Your World with Food! by John Robbins

Diet for a New America: How Your Food Choices Affect Your Health, Happiness and the Future of Life on Earth (2nd edition) by John Robbins

No Happy Cows: Dispatches from the Frontlines of the Food Revolution by John Robbins

The Food Revolution: How Your Diet Can Help Save Your Life and Our World by John Robbins

The Restore-Our-Planet Diet: Food Choice, Our Environment, and Our Heath by Patricia Tallman, PhD

COOKBOOKS

Dr. Neal Barnard's Cookbook for Reversing Diabetes: 150 Recipes Scientifically Proven to Reverse Diabetes Without Drugs by Dr. Neal Barnard

The Get Healthy, Go Vegan Cookbook: 125 Easy and Delicious Recipes to Jump-Start Weight Loss and Help You Feel Great by Dr. Neal Barnard

The How Not to Die Cookbook: 100+ Recipes to Help Prevent and Reverse Disease by Dr. Michael Greger

The McDougall Quick and Easy Cookbook: Over 300 Delicious Low-Fat Recipes You Can Prepare in Fifteen Minutes or Less by Dr. John McDougall

PETA's Vegan College Cookbook by PETA

LIFESTYLE CHANGES

The Mason Jar Cookbook: 80 Healthy and Portable Meals by Amy Fazio

Waste-Free Kitchen Handbook: A Guide to Eating Well and Saving Money by Wasting Less Food by Dana Gunders

Zero Waste Home: The Ultimate Guide to Simplifying Your Life by Reducing Your Waste by Bea Johnson

DOCUMENTARIES/TV

Devour the Earth

Eating You Alive

Forks Over Knives

The Game Changers

Merchants of Doubt

A Plastic Ocean

What the Health

Years of Living Dangerously

WEBSITES

Environmental Working Group: www.ewg.org/meateatersguide/

American College of Lifestyle Medicine: www.lifestylemedicine.org

Earth Guardians: www.earthguardians.org

Forks Over Knives: www.forksoverknives.com

Local Harvest CSA Locator: www.localharvest.org/csa/

NutritionFacts.org (Dr. Michael Greger): nutritionfacts.org

One Green Planet: www.forksoverknives.comonegreenplanet.org

Physician's Committee for Responsible Medicine (Dr. Neal Barnard): www.pcrm.org and www.pcrm.org/health/diets/kickstart

The 200 Year Project: www.200yearproject.com

Two Zesty Bananas: www.twozestybananas.com

Vegan Society (UK): www.vegansociety.com

Vegetarian Nutrition Dietetic Practice Group of the (Academy of Nutrition and Dietetics): vegetariannutrition.net

Vegetarian Resource Group: www.vrg.org/nutrition/

BLOGS (a great source of recipes!)

Deliciously Ella: deliciouslyella.com

Hot for Food: www.hotforfoodblog.com/welcome

Keepin' It Kind: keepinitkind.com

Oh She Glows: ohsheglows.com

Plant-Based Dietitian: plantbaseddietitian.com

Sprouted Kitchen: www.sproutedkitchen.com

Trinity's Conscious Kitchen: www.trinityskitchen.com

The Vegan 8: thevegan8.com

The Vegan RD: www.theveganrd.com

Acknowledgments

We are on a wild ride. And this book is an important piece of my life's greater mission—to take care of the planet and make the world a better place for all our children—a mission that has expanded and grown over the years thanks to the hard work, passion, and commitment of many people. This movement has always been about collective effort toward a greater cause, and this book is certainly no exception.

The person who is responsible for propelling us into the plant-based world is Elliot Washor for suggesting we watch *Forks Over Knives* nine months before we finally got around to it, on May 7, 2012.

Then OMD all began with my brother-in-law, Jeff King, saying at MUSE School, "It's only one meal a day, people!" and a seed was planted! MUSE has been an enormous part of my growth. My sister Rebecca Amis has been shoulder to shoulder with me, and I'm so deeply grateful to her and Jeff. Also, thank you to all of the children and families at MUSE, along with Team MUSE, for doing OMD every day.

My Amis family roots are strong and enduring. Thanks to my mother for vegan creamed corn, and who taught me discipline and tenacity, my daddy who taught me to believe in myself, and my sisters and brothers who keep me honest and remind me where I come from.

Toward the creation of the book, I'd like to thank my agent Heather Jackson, Mariska van Aalst, the gracious and devoted Sarah Pelz, and a host of people at Atria who make this all possible. Thank you to Dr. Alfredo Mejia in the Environmental Nutrition group of the Department of Public Health, Nutrition, and Wellness at Andrews University for helping us measure the environmental impact savings for each of our recipes.

For those in our "brain trust" who have contributed to the book through their inspiration, teaching, books, counsel and assistance, I'd like to thank Dr. Dean Ornish, Dr. Neal Barnard, Samuel Lee-Gammage, Dr. T. Colin Campbell, Kathy Freston, Tal Ronnen, Dr. Caldwell and Rip Esselstyn, Dr. Michael Greger, Dr. John McDougall, Renee Lertzman, Moby, Arianna Huffington, Maria Shriver, Christiana Musk, Maria Wilhelm, Mathew Kinney, Jessica Alba, Jonathan Robbins, Francis Moore Lappe, Ocean Robbins, Rich Roll, Dr. Jay Gordon, Richard Oppenlander, Jim Morris Hicks, Craig McCaw, Stephen Leahy, and to the organizations working tirelessly to make the world a better place: Physicians Committee for Responsible Medicine, Climate Nexus, Friends of the Earth, Chef Ann Foundation, Sierra Club, Earth Guardians, Center for Biological Diversity, Good Food Institute, Greenpeace, Better Buying Lab, Food Climate Research Network, Chatham House, Real Food Challenge, Meatless Mondays, The Center for Good Food Purchasing, One Green Planet, Earth Justice.

And thank you to all of those who contributed their stories, Dame Patsy Reddy, Sir David Gascoigne, Ken Beatty, Davien Littlefield, Allison Braine, Jenny Briesch, Chrissy and Stuart Bullard, Zoe Nachum, Elle Tortorici, Sarah Jones, Brian Theiss, and the many, many who have shared their stories with us along the way.

For the OMD movement-building, the campaign work on healthy school lunch programs, the restaurant work, and so many other things, I'd like to thank Ashley Schaeffer-Yildiz, Jessica Jewell-Lanier, and Maggie Taylor. Karen Bouris keeps it all together, along with Paulo, Amelia, Cindy, and so many others.

To my children Jasper, Soli, Josa, Claire, Quinn, and Rose.

And finally, to Jim, my partner in all things.

Notes

CHAPTER 1: OUR OMD JOURNEY

1   M. Song, T. T. Fung, F. B. Hu, et al., "Association of Animal and Plant Protein Intake With All-Cause and Cause-Specific Mortality," *JAMA Internal Medicine* 176, no. 10 (October 1, 2016): 1453–1463.

2   P. N. Singh, J. Sabaté, and G. E. Fraser, "Does Low Meat Consumption Increase Life Expectancy in Humans?" *American Journal of Clinical Nutrition* 78, suppl. 3 (September 1, 2003): 526S–532S.

3   F. L. Crowe, P. N. Appleby, R. C. Travis, et al., "Risk of hospitalization or death from ischemic heart disease among British vegetarians and nonvegetarians: results from the EPIC-Oxford cohort study," *American Journal of Clinical Nutrition* 97, no. 3 (March 1, 2013): 597–603.

4   S. Tonstad, K. Stewart, K. Oda, et al., "Vegetarian diets and incidence of diabetes in the Adventist Health Study 2," *Nutrition, Metabolism, and Cardiovascular Disease* 23, no. 4 (April 2013): 292–9.

5   Y. Tantamango-Bartley, K. Jaceldo-Siegl, J. Fan, et al., "Vegetarian diets and the incidence of cancer in a low-risk population," *Cancer Epidemiology, Biomarkers & Prevention* 22, no. 2 (February 2013): 286–94.

6   N. D. Barnard, A. I. Bush, A. Ceccarelli, et al., "Dietary and lifestyle guidelines for the prevention of Alzheimer's disease," *Neurobiology of Aging* 35, suppl. 2 (September 2014): S74–8.

CHAPTER 2: OMD FOR YOUR HEALTH

1   J. Hever, "Plant-Based Diets: A Physician's Guide," *Permanente Journal* 20, no. 3 (Summer 2016): 93–101.

2   M. Rosell, P. Appleby, E. Spencer, et al., "Weight gain over 5 years in 21,966 meat-eating, fish-eating, vegetarian, and vegan men and women in EPIC-Oxford," *International Journal of Obesity* (London) 30, no. 9 (September 2006): 1389–96.

3   H. R. Ferdowsian and N. D. Barnard, "Effects of plant-based diets on plasma lipids," *American Journal of Cardiology* 104, no. 7 (October 1, 2009): 947–56.

4   A. J. Lanou and B. Svenson, "Reduced cancer risk in vegetarians: an analysis of
    recent reports," *Cancer Management and Research* 3 (December 20, 2010): 1–8.

5   H. R. Ferdowsian and N. D. Barnard, "Effects of plant-based diets on plasma
    lipids," *American Journal of Cardiology* 104, no. 7 (October 1, 2009): 947–56.

6   P. N. Appleby, G. K. Davey, and T. J. Key, "Hypertension and blood pressure
    among meat eaters, fish eaters, vegetarians and vegans in EPIC-Oxford," *Public
    Health Nutrition* 5, no. 5 (December 2002): 645–54.

7   S. Tonstad, T. Butler, R. Yan, et al., "Type of vegetarian diet, body weight, and
    prevalence of type 2 diabetes," *Diabetes Care* 32, no. 5 (May 2009): 791–6.

8   M. J. Orlich, P. N. Singh, J. Sabaté, et al., "Vegetarian dietary patterns and
    mortality in Adventist Health Study 2." *JAMA Internal Medicine* 173, no. 13
    (July 8, 2013): 1230–8.

9   Orlich et al, "Vegetarian dietary patterns and mortality."

10 D. Ornish, "Statins and the soul of medicine," *American Journal of Cardiology*
    89, no. 11 (June 1, 2002): 1286–90; D. J. Jenkins, C. W. Kendall, A. Marchie,
    et al., "Direct comparison of a dietary portfolio of cholesterol-lowering foods
    with a statin in hypercholesterolemic participants," *American Journal of
    Clinical Nutrition* 81, no. 2 (February 2005): 380–7; N. D. Barnard, J. Cohen,
    D. J. Jenkins, et al., "A low-fat vegan diet and a conventional diabetes diet in the
    treatment of type 2 diabetes: a randomized, controlled, 74-wk clinical trial,"
    American Journal of Clinical Nutrition 89, no. 5 (May 2009): 1588S–1596S.
    https://www.ncbi.nlm.nih.gov/pubmed/19339401.

11 D. Ornish, L. W. Scherwitz, J. H. Billings, et al., "Intensive lifestyle changes for
    reversal of coronary heart disease," *JAMA* 280, no. 23 (December 16, 1998):
    2001–7.

12 C. B. Esselstyn Jr., G. Gendy, J. Doyle, et al., "A way to reverse CAD?" *Journal of
    Family Practice* 63, no. 7 (July 2014): 356–364b.

13 Barnard et al., "A low-fat vegan diet."

14 D. Tilman and M. Clark, "Global Diets Link Environmental Sustainability and
    Human Health," *Nature* 515 (November 27, 2014): 518–22.

15 R. A. Koeth, Z. Wang, B. S. Levison, et al., "Intestinal microbiota metabolism of
    L-carnitine, a nutrient in red meat, promotes atherosclerosis," *Natural Medicine
    Journal* 19, no. 5 (May 2013): 576–85.

16 H. C. Hung, K. J. Joshipura, R. Jiang, et al., "Fruit and vegetable intake and risk
    of major chronic disease," *Journal of the National Cancer Institute* 96, no. 21
    (November 3, 2004): 1577–84.

17 P. Tuso, S. R. Stoll, and W. W. Li, "A Plant-Based Diet, Atherogenesis, and
    Coronary Artery Disease Prevention," *Permanente Journal* 19, no. 1 (2015):
    62–67.

18 D. Ornish, S. E. Brown, L. W. Scherwitz, et al., "Can lifestyle changes reverse coronary heart disease? The Lifestyle Heart Trial," *Lancet* 336, no. 8708 (July 21, 1990): 129–33.

19 Ornish et al., "Intensive lifestyle changes."

20 K. M. Adams, K. C. Lindell, M. Kohlmeier, et al., "Status of nutrition education in medical schools," *American Journal of Clinical Nutrition* 83, no. 4 (April 2006): 941S–944S. https://academic.oup.com/ajcn/article/83/4/941S/4649273.

21 https://www.cdc.gov/diabetes/pdfs/data/statistics/national-diabetes-statistics -report.pdf.

22 A. Pan, Q. Sun, A. M. Bernstein, et al., "Changes in red meat consumption and subsequent risk of type 2 diabetes mellitus: three cohorts of US men and women," *JAMA Internal Medicine* 173, no. 14 (July 22, 2013): 1328–35.

23 M. Knip and O. Simell, "Environmental triggers of type 1 diabetes," *Cold Spring Harbor Perspectives in Medicine* 2, no. 7 (July 2012): a007690.

24 D. A. Snowdon and R. L. Phillips, "Does a vegetarian diet reduce the occurrence of diabetes?" *American Journal of Public Health* 75, no. 5 (May 1985): 507–12.

25 A. Vang, P. N. Singh, J. W. Lee, et al., "Meats, processed meats, obesity, weight gain and occurrence of diabetes among adults: findings from Adventist Health Studies," *Annals of Nutrition and Metabolism* 52, no. 2 (2008): 96–104.

26 N. D. Barnard, J. Cohen, D. J. Jenkins, et al., "A low-fat vegan diet improves glycemic control and cardiovascular risk factors in a randomized clinical trial in individuals with type 2 diabetes," *Diabetes Care* 29, no. 8 (August 2006): 1777–83.

27 H. Kahleova, M. Klementova, V. Herynek, et al., "The Effect of a Vegetarian vs. Conventional Hypocaloric Diabetic Diet on Thigh Adipose Tissue Distribution in Subjects with Type 2 Diabetes: A Randomized Study," *Journal of the American College of Nutrition* 36, no. 5 (July 2017): 364–69.

28 A. Nehra, "Erectile dysfunction and cardiovascular disease: efficacy and safety of phosphodiesterase type 5 inhibitors in men with both conditions," *Mayo Clinic Proceedings* 84, no. 2 (February 2009): 139–48.

29 G. Bennett and F. Williams, *Mainstream Green: Moving Sustainability from Niche to Normal* (Ogilvy & Mather, 2011) accessed from https://madeleineporr .files.wordpress.com/2018/03/2011-mainstream_green.pdf.

30 M. B. Ruby and S. J. Heine, "Meat, morals, and masculinity," *Appetite* 56, no. 2 (April 2011): 447–50.

31 C. Eleazu, N. Obianuju, K. Eleaz, et al., "The role of dietary polyphenols in the management of erectile dysfunction-Mechanisms of action," *Biomedicine & Pharmacotherapy* 88 (April 2017): 644–52.

32 S. E. Berkow and N. D. Barnard, "Vegetarian diets and weight status," *Nutrition Reviews* 64, no. 4 (April 2006): 175–88.

33 N. S. Rizzo, K. Jaceldo-Siegl, J. Sabaté, et al., "Nutrient profiles of vegetarian and nonvegetarian dietary patterns," *Journal of the Academy of Nutrition and Dietetics* 113, no. 12 (December 2013): 1610–9.

34 M. Rosell, P. Appleby, E. Spencer, et al., "Weight gain over 5 years in 21,966 meat-eating, fish-eating, vegetarian, and vegan men and women in EPIC-Oxford," *International Journal of Obesity* (London) 30, no. 9 (September 2006): 1389–96.

35 J. Sabaté and W. Wien, "Vegetarian diets and childhood obesity prevention," *American Journal of Clinical Nutrition* 91, no. 5 (May 2010): 1525S–1529S. https://www.ncbi.nlm.nih.gov/pubmed/20237136.

36 B. Farmer, B. T. Larson, V. L. Fulgoni III, et al., "A vegetarian dietary pattern as a nutrient-dense approach to weight management: an analysis of the national health and nutrition examination survey 1999–2004," *Journal of the American Dietetic Association* 111, no. 6 (June 2011): 819–27.

37 N. E. Allen, P. N. Appleby, G. K. Davey, et al., "The associations of diet with serum insulin-like growth factor I and its main binding proteins in 292 women meat-eaters, vegetarians, and vegans," *Cancer Epidemiology, Biomarkers & Prevention* 11, no. 11 (November 2002): 1441–8.

38 N. M. Bastide, F. H. Pierre, and D. E. Corpet, "Heme iron from meat and risk of colorectal cancer: a meta-analysis and a review of the mechanisms involved," *Cancer Prevention Research* (Philadelphia) 4, no. 2 (February 2011): 177–84.

39 C. Dall, "FDA: Antibiotic use in food animals continues to rise," Center for Infectious Disease Research and Policy, University of Minnesota. December 22, 2016.

40 M. P. Francino, "Antibiotics and the Human Gut Microbiome: Dysbioses and Accumulation of Resistances," *Frontiers in Microbiology* 12, no. 6 (January 2016): 1543.

41 L. Guthrie, S. Gupta, J. Daily, and L. Kelly, "Human microbiome signatures of differential colorectal cancer drug metabolism," *npj Biofilms Microbiomes* 1, no. 3 (November 2017): 27.

42 P. N. Appleby, F. L. Crowe, K. E. Bradbury, et al., "Mortality in vegetarians and comparable nonvegetarians in the United Kingdom," *American Journal of Clinical Nutrition* 103, no.1 (2016): 218–230. http://doi.org/10.3945/ajcn .115.119461.

43 Y. Tantamango-Bartley, K. Jaceldo-Siegl, J. Fan, and G. Fraser, "Vegetarian diets and the incidence of cancer in a low-risk population," *Cancer Epidemiology, Biomarkers & Prevention* 22, no. 2 (February 2013): 286–94.

44 "Phytochemicals: The Cancer Fighters in Your Foods," American Institute for Cancer Research. www.aicr.org/reduce-your-cancer-risk/diet/elements _phytochemicals.html.

45 K. S. Bishop and L. R. Ferguson, "The interaction between epigenetics, nutrition and the development of cancer," *Nutrients* 7, no. 2 (January 30, 2015): 922–47.

46 S. A. Kim, L. V. Moore, D. Galuska, et al., "Vital Signs: Fruit and Vegetable Intake Among Children—United States, 2003–2010," *Mortality and Morbidity Weekly Report* 63, no. 31 (2014): 671–76. http://www.cdc.gov/mmwr/preview /mmwrhtml/mm6331a3.htm?s_cid=mm6331a3_w.

47 I. Nathan, A. F. Hackett, and S. Kirby, "A longitudinal study of the growth of matched pairs of vegetarian and omnivorous children, aged 7–11 years, in the northwest of England," *European Journal of Clinical Nutrition* 51, no. 1 (1997): 20–25.

48 C. E. Yen, C. H. Yen, M. C. Huang, C. H. Cheng, and Y. C. Huang, "Dietary intake and nutritional status of vegetarian and omnivorous preschool children and their parents in Taiwan," *Nutrition Research* (New York, NY) 28, no. 7 (2008): 430–6.

49 J. T. Dwyer, L. G. Miller, N. L. Arduino, et al., "Mental age and I.Q. of predominately vegetarian children," *Journal of the American Dietetic Association* 76 (1980): 142–7.

50 C. R. Gale, I. J. Deary, G. Batty, and I. Schoon, "IQ in childhood and vegetarianism in adulthood: 1970 British cohort study," *BMJ* 334 (2007): 245–8.

51 P. Giem, W. L. Beeson, and G. E. Fraser, "The incidence of dementia and intake of animal products: Preliminary findings from the Adventist Health Study," *Neuroepidemiology* 12, no. 1 (1993): 28–36.

52 M. C. Morris, D. A. Evans, J. L. Bienias, et al., "Dietary fats and the risk of incident Alzheimer disease," *Archives of Neurology* 60 (2003): 194–200.

53 M. C. Morris, D. A. Evans, J. L. Bienias, et al., "Dietary intake of antioxidant nutrients and the risk of incident Alzheimer disease in a biracial community study," *JAMA* 287 (2002): 3230–7.

54 E. E. Devore, F. Grodstein, F. J. van Rooij, et al., "Dietary antioxidants and long-term risk of dementia," *Archives of Neurology* 67 (2010): 819–25.

55 E. Ernst, L. Pietsch, A. Matrai, and J. Eisenberg, "Blood rheology in vegetarians," *British Journal of Nutrition* 56, no. 3 (1986): 555–60.

56 J. Piazza, M. B. Ruby, S. Loughnan, et al., "Rationalizing meat consumption. The 4Ns," *Appetite* 91 (August 2015): 114–28.

57 M. Song, T. T. Fung, F. B. Hu, et al., "Association of Animal and Plant Protein Intake With All-Cause and Cause-Specific Mortality," *JAMA Internal Medicine* 176, no. 10 (October 1, 2016): 1453–63.

58 D. Ornish, J. Lin, J. M. Chan, et al., "Effect of comprehensive lifestyle changes on telomerase activity and telomere length in men with biopsy-proven low-risk prostate cancer: 5-year follow-up of a descriptive pilot study," *Lancet Oncology* 14, no. 11 (October 2013): 1112–20.

59 P. N. Singh, J. Sabaté, and G. E. Fraser, "Does low meat consumption increase life expectancy in humans?" *American Journal of Clinical Nutrition* 78, suppl. 3 (September 2003): 526S–532S.

CHAPTER 3: OMD FOR THE PLANET

1 https://www.epa.gov/ghgemissions/understanding-global-warming-potentials.

2 https://www.ipcc.ch/pdf/assessment-report/ar5/wg1/WG1AR5_Chapter08_FINAL.pdf.

3 https://www.theguardian.com/environment/2016/mar/21/eat-less-meat-vegetarianism-dangerous-global-warming.

4 https://www.chathamhouse.org/sites/files/chathamhouse/field/field_document/20141203LivestockClimateChangeForgottenSectorBaileyFroggatt WellesleyFinal.pdf.

5 B. Bajželj, et al. Importance of food-demand management for climate mitigation, *Nature Climate Change* 4 (2014): 924-29.

6 http://nca2014.globalchange.gov/highlights#section-5681.

7 https://19january2017snapshot.epa.gov/climate-impacts/international-climate-impacts_.html.

8 https://www.nature.com/articles/s41598-017-04134-5.

9 https://news.nationalgeographic.com/2017/07/sea-level-rise-flood-global-warming-science/.

10 http://ucsusa.maps.arcgis.com/apps/MapSeries/index.html?appid=64b2cbd03a3d4b87aaddaf65f6b33332.

11 https://www.epa.gov/ghgemissions/understanding-global-warming-potentials.

12 S. Stoll-Kleemann and T. O'Riordan, "The Sustainability Challenges of Our Meat and Dairy Diets," *Environment* 57, no. 2 (April 23, 2015): 34–48.

13 http://www.fao.org/3/a-i3437e.pdf.

14 https://www.chathamhouse.org/sites/files/ chathamhouse/field/field_document/20141203LivestockClimateChangeForgottenSectorBaileyFroggatt WellesleyFinal.pdf.

15 http://www.fao.org/ag/againfo/resources/en/publications/tackling_climate_change/index.htm.

16 https://www.pri.org/stories/2017-10-30/theres-more-co2-atmosphere-now-any-point-almost-million-years.

17 https://climate.nasa.gov/vital-signs/arctic-sea-ice/.

18 http://ocean.si.edu/sea-level-rise.

19 https://www.smithsonianmag.com/science-nature/beef-uses-ten-times-more
-resources-poultry-dairy-eggs-pork-180952103/.

20 https://globalforestatlas.yale.edu/land-use/industrial-agriculture.

21 http://www.fao.org/3/a-i5588e.pdf.

22 https://globalforestatlas.yale.edu/amazon/land-use/cattle-ranching.

23 G. Koneswaran, D. Nierenberg, "Global farm animal production and global
warming: impacting and mitigating climate change," Environ Health Perspect.
(May 2008); 116(5): 578–82.

24 https://www.youtube.com/watch?v=ysa5OBhXz-Q.

25 https://www.nature.com/articles/nature10452.

26 http://science.sciencemag.org/content/343/6167/1241484.

27 http://www.pbl.nl/en/publications/2011/meat-dairy-and-fish-options-for
-changes-in-production-and-consumption.

28 http://www.wri.org/blog/2016/04/sustainable-diets-what-you-need-know-12
-charts.

29 https://www.ucsusa.org/our-work/food-agriculture/our-failing-food-system
/industrial-agriculture#.Wj2oSlQ-eji.

30 https://www.scientificamerican.com/article/Earth-talks-daily-destruction/.

31 http://science.sciencemag.org/content/321/5891/926.

32 http://www.noaa.gov/media-release/gulf-of-mexico-dead-zone-is-largest-ever
-measured.

33 http://siteresources.worldbank.org/INTENVMAT/Resources/3011340
-1238620444756/5980735-1238620476358/13ECA.pdf.

34 P. Scarborough, P. N. Appleby, A. Mizdrak, et al., "Dietary greenhouse gas
emissions of meat-eaters, fish-eaters, vegetarians and vegans in the UK,"
Climatic Change 125, no. 2 (2014): 179–92.

35 https://www.pbs.org/newshour/science/the-hidden-costs-of-hamburgers.

36 https://www.smithsonianmag.com/science-nature/beef-uses-ten-times-more
-resources-poultry-dairy-eggs-pork-180952103/.

37 https://ourworldindata.org/meat-and-seafood-production-consumption.

38 https://climatenexus.org/climate-change-news/chinese-officials-join-forces
-with-american-celebrities-urging-sharp-cut-in-meat-consumption/.

39 K. Gee, "America's Dairy Farmers Dump 43 Million Gallons of Excess Milk,"
Wall Street Journal, October 12, 2016.

40 https://www.bloomberg.com/news/features/2017-07-19/the-mad-cheese
-scientists-fighting-to-save-the-dairy-industry.

41 http://www.businessinsider.com/the-35-companies-that-spent-1-billion-on
-ads-in-2011-2012-11.

42 Immanuel Ness. *Encyclopedia of National Interest Groups*, Routledge (July
2015): 233.

43 https://www.agweb.com/article/contemporary_beef_marketing_campaign
_builds_on_popular_successful_tagline_naa_news_release/.

44 https://www.opensecrets.org/industries/background.php?cycle=2014&ind=
G2300.

45 Per Dr. Barnard, private communication, 4/2018.

46 https://www.ers.usda.gov/data-products/dairy-data/.

47 http://www.mintel.com/press-centre/food-and-drink/us-sales-of-dairy-milk
-turn-sour-as-non-dairy-milk-sales-grow-9-in-2015.

48 http://ir.tyson.com/investor-relations/news-releases/news-releases-details/2016
/Beyond-Meat-and-Tyson-Foods-Announce-Investment-Agreement/default
.aspx.

49 http://ir.tyson.com/investor-relations/news-releases/news-releases-details
/2017/Tyson-Foods-Makes-Additional-Investment-in-Beyond-Meat/default
.aspx.

50 J. Macy and M. Young Brown, "Coming Back to Life" (British Columbia,
Canada: New Society Publishers, 1998).

CHAPTER 4: PREPARE TO OMD

1 https://www.chathamhouse.org/sites/files/chathamhouse/field/field_
document/20141203LivestockClimateChangeForgottenSectorBaileyFroggatt
WellesleyFinal.pdf.

2 M. Guasch-Ferré, X. Liu, V. S. Malik, et al., "Nut Consumption and Risk of
Cardiovascular Disease," *Journal of the American College of Cardiology* 70,
no. 20 (November 2017): 2519–2532.

3 G. Eshel, A. Shepon, T. Makov, and R. Milo, "Land, irrigation water,
greenhouse gas, and reactive nitrogen burdens of meat, eggs, and dairy
production in the United States," *PNAS* 111, no. 33 (August 19, 2014): 11996–
12001.

4 https://www.cdc.gov/foodborneburden/attribution-1998-2008.html.

5 S. Park, S. Navratil, A. Gregory, et al., "Generic *Escherichia coli* contamination
of spinach at the preharvest stage: effects of farm management and
environmental factors," *Applied and Environmental Microbiology* 79, no. 14
(July 2013): 4347–58.

6 https://epha.org/animal-farming-public-health-unavoidable-transition
-towards-sustainable-healthy-diets/.

7   A. Y. Kamila, "Eating less meat can make a real difference in fighting climate change," *Portland Press Herald*, February 1, 2017.

8   S. Clune et al., "Systematic review of greenhouse gas emissions for different fresh food categories," *Journal of Cleaner Production* 140, part 2 (January 1, 2017): 766–83.

9   S. Tonstad, T. Butler, R. Yan, G. E. Fraser, "Type of vegetarian diet, body weight and prevalence of type 2 diabetes," *Diabetes Care* 32, no. 5 (2009): 791–6.

10 "Position of the Academy of Nutrition and Dietetics: Vegetarian Diets," *Journal of the Academy of Nutrition and Dietetics* 116 (2016): 1970–80.

11 P. N. Appleby and T. J. Key, "The long-term health of vegetarians and vegans," *Proceedings of the Nutrition Society* 75 (2016): 287–93.

12 L. T. Le and J. Sabaté, "Beyond meatless, the health effects of vegan diets: findings from the Adventist cohorts," *Nutrients* 6, no. 6 (May 27, 2014): 2131–47.

13 http://www.nationalacademies.org/hmd/~/media/Files/Activity%20Files/Nutrition/DRI-Tables/5Summary%20TableTables%2014.pdf?la=en.

14 R. Pawlak, et al., "The prevalence of cobalamin deficiency among vegetarians assessed by serum vitamin B_{12}: a review of literature," *European Journal of Clinical Nutrition* (2014) 68: 541–8.

15 D. Rogerson, "Vegan diets: practical advice for athletes and exercisers," *Journal of the International Society of Sports Nutrition* 14 (2017): 36.

16 W. S. Harris, "Achieving optimal n-3 fatty acid status: the vegetarian's challenge . . . or not," *American Journal of Clinical Nutrition* 100, suppl. (2014): 449S–52S.

17 https://nccih.nih.gov/health/omega3/introduction.htm#hed6.

18 A. V. Saunders, B. C. Davis, M. L. Garg, "Omega-3 polyunsaturated fatty acids and vegetarian diets," *Medical Journal of Australia* 199, suppl. 4 (2013): 22S–26S.

19 H. Watanabe, "Beneficial biological effects of miso with reference to radiation injury, cancer and hypertension," *Journal of Toxicologic Pathology* 26, no. 2 (June 2013): 91–103.

20 J. Kern, S. Kern, K. Blennow, et al., "Calcium supplementation and risk of dementia in women with cerebrovascular disease," *Neurology* 87, no. 16 (October 18, 2016): 1674–80.

21 J. J. Anderson, B. Kruszka, J. A. Delaney, et al., "Calcium Intake From Diet and Supplements and the Risk of Coronary Artery Calcification and its Progression Among Older Adults: 10-Year Follow-up of the Multi-Ethnic Study of Atherosclerosis (MESA)," *Journal of the American Heart Association* 5, no. 10 (October 11, 2016).

22 S. Van Vliet et al., "The Skeletal Muscle Anabolic Response to Plant- versus Animal-Based Protein Consumption," *Journal of Nutrition* 145 (2015): 1981–91.

23 M. G. Nosworthy et al., "Effect of Processing on the *in Vitro* and *in Vivo* Protein Quality of Yellow and Green Split Peas (*Pisum sativum*)," *Journal of Agricultural and Food Chemistry* 65, no. 35 (2017): 7790–6.

24 X. O. Shu, Y. Zheng, H. Cai, et al., "Soy food intake and breast cancer survival," *JAMA* 302, no. 22 (December 9, 2009): 2437–43.

25 L. Yan and E. L. Spitznagel, "Soy consumption and prostate cancer risk in men: a revisit of a meta-analysis," *American Journal of Clinical Nutrition* 89, no. 4 (April 2009): 1155–63.

26 K. Michaëlsson, A. Wolk, S. Langenskiöld, et al., "Milk intake and risk of mortality and fractures in women and men: cohort studies," *BMJ* 349 (October 28, 2014): g6015.

27 A. Bouzari et al., "Vitamin retention in eight fruits and vegetables: a comparison of refrigerated and frozen storage," *Journal of Agricultural and Food Chemistry* 63, no. 3 (January 28, 2015): 957–62.

28 A. Bouzari et al., "Mineral, fiber, and total phenolic retention in eight fruits and vegetables: a comparison of refrigerated and frozen storage," *Journal of Agricultural and Food Chemistry* 63, no. 3 (January 28, 2015): 951–6.

29 C. M. G. C. Renard et al., "Home conservation strategies for tomato (Solanum lycopersicum): Storage temperature vs. duration—Is there a compromise for better aroma preservation?" *Food Chemistry* 139 (2013): 825–36.

30 L. Fisher and L. Medeiros, "Refrigerator Storage," Ohioline, Ohio State University Extension. https://ohioline.osu.edu/factsheet/HYG-5403.

31 Penn State Extension: https://extension.psu.edu/buying-guide-fruit.

32 US Highbush Blueberry Council, "Buying Blueberries," https://www.blueberrycouncil.org/blueberry-cooking-tips/buying-blueberries/; Grapes from California, "All About Grapes," https://www.grapesfromcalifornia.com/all-about-grapes/.

33 Fisher and Medeiros, "Refrigerator Storage."

34 Florida Department of Citrus, "How Long will fresh Florida Grapefruit keep in the fridge?," https://www.floridacitrus.org/grapefruit/facts.

35 Hale Groves, "How to Find the Best Grapefruit Year Round," http://blog.halegroves.com/how-to-find-the-best-grapefruit-year-round/.

36 Georgia Peach Council, "Choosing and Processing Peaches," http://gapeaches.org/recipes/choosing-and-processing-peaches/.

37 California Strawberry Commission, "Select and Store," http://www.californiastrawberries.com/about/select-and-store/.

38 Fisher and Medeiros, "Refrigerator Storage."

39 Penn State Extension, "Buying Guide: Vegetables," https://extension.psu.edu/buying-guide-vegetables.

40 N. Hedstrom, "Bulletin #4177, Vegetables and Fruits for Health: Broccoli and Cauliflower," University of Maine Extension, https://extension.umaine.edu /publications/4177e/.

41 J. McGarry, "The fantastic health benefits of kale," Michigan State University Extension, 2014, http://msue.anr.msu.edu/news/the_fantastic_health_benefits _of_kale.

42 K. Savoie and K. Yerxa, "Bulletin #4180, Vegetables and Fruits for Health: Greens," University of Maine Extension, https://extension.umaine.edu /publications/4180e/.

CHAPTER 5: ONE MEAL A DAY

1 H. Harwatt, J. Sabaté, G. Eshel, et al., "Substituting beans for beef as a contribution toward US climate change targets," *Climatic Change* 143, 1–2 (July 2017): 261–70. Chapter 6: All-In

1 H. Fields, D. Millstine, N. Agrwal, L. Marks, "Is Meat Killing Us?," *Journal of the American Osteopathic Association* 116, no. 5 (May 1, 2016): 296–300.

2 https://www.consumerreports.org/cro/magazine/2015/01/how-much-arsenic -is-in-your-rice/index.htm.

3 https://nutritionfacts.org/2016/03/22/the-effects-of-dietary-cholesterol-on -blood-cholesterol/.

4 https://scienmag.com/study-finds-consuming-nuts-strengthens-brainwave -function/.

CHAPTER 8: YOUR TIME TO SHINE

1 https://www.washingtonpost.com/lifestyle/food/in-la-vegetables-are-the-stars /2017/03/31/9d6bc6fa-13e8-11e7-ada0-1489b735b3a3_story.html.

2 http://www.supermarketnews.com/consumer-trends/future-plant-based-foods.

3 https://www.chathamhouse.org/sites/files/chathamhouse/field/field _document/20141203LivestockClimateChangeForgottenSectorBaileyFroggatt WellesleyFinal.pdf.

Index

A

afternoon tea, 159–60
aging, 9, 60, 185
All-In, 170, 171–98
  benefits of, 173–74
  as choice, 196–98
  14-day menu plan, 187–95
  14-day menu plan shopping list, 305–12
  mind tricks for, 178–79
  toolkit for, 179–83
  in two jumps, 174–75
almond milk, 121–22, 124, 125, 214–15
almonds, 103
  Ree Ree's Raw Vegan Taco Nut "Meat," 226–27
alpha-linolenic acid (ALA), 53, 111–13
Alzheimer's disease and dementia, 9
Amazon Basin, 72
American Diabetes Association, 36–37
American Journal of Clinical Nutrition, 43, 60
amino acids, 52, 117
Amis, Rebecca, xi–xii, 6, 7, 13, 14, 16, 50, 226, 241
Andrews University, 184
animal agriculture, 47–48, 57, 62–63, 286, 288–89
  biodiversity and, 73–75
  climate change and, 11, 49–50, 62, 65–66, 69–71, 81
  dead zones and, 75–76
  food safety and, 100–101
  forests and, xviii, 11, 73
  water usage and, xviii, 11, 76–77
animal products, 40, 50
  protein in, xv, xvi, 16, 30
  see also dairy; meat, meat-based diet
antibiotics, 47–48, 49, 100, 101, 179
antioxidants, 32–33, 49
apples:
  applesauce, 233
  Ben's Apple-Walnut "Mouffins," 213–14
arsenic, 183–84
Asparagus and Sun-Dried Tomato Lasagna, Brad and Sandy's, 250–52
athletes, 43, 53, 117
Avatar, 11, 12, 72, 142, 250, 286

B

B_{12}, 110–11
Barnard, Neal, 16, 23, 26, 36–37, 43–44, 51, 96, 173, 174–75, 180, 181
beans, 233–34
  Basic Black Beans, 224–25
  Food Forest Organics Burgers, 238–39
  Open-Faced Peppers, 239–40
  soaking, 157
  Suzy's Family Favorite Chili, 230
Beatty, Ken, 44–46
Beatty, Page, 42, 44
beef, xviii, 23, 31, 47, 56, 71, 73–75, 82, 84, 102
  burgers, 73, 74, 76–78, 83, 141–42, 147, 173, 286
  organic grass-fed, 7, 39, 50, 143
bees, 163–64
biodiversity, 73–75
Biomedicine & Pharmacology, 38
Bittman, Mark, 169

Blackburn, Elizabeth, 59
blood flow, xvi, 53
blood pressure, xvii, 26, 30, 38, 53, 173
Blueberry-Lemon-Coconut Scones,
    211–12
brain, xv–xvi, 52
Braine, Allison, 54–55
breakfast recipes, 201–14
Briesch, Jenny, 104–5
British Medical Journal, 123
Bullard, Chrissy and Stuart, 144–45
burgers, beef, 73, 74, 76–78, 83,
    141–42, 147, 173, 286
Burgers, Food Forest Organics,
    238–39

C
cabbage:
    BBQ "Chicken" Sliders with Classic
        Coleslaw, 236–37
    Soli and Jasper's Curtido, 245–46
cake:
    Dark Chocolate Lamington Cakes
        with Blackberry Sorbet, 270–73
    Suzy's Carrot Cake, 275–76
calcium, 114–15, 116, 117
Cameron, James, xx, 6–14, 27, 35, 37,
    39, 42, 44, 45, 62, 64, 72, 86,
    147–48, 179, 181, 183, 185, 196,
    197, 286, 287, 289
    DEEPSEA CHALLENGE
        Expedition of, 69–70
Cameron, Suzy Amis, 3–13
Cameron Family Farms, xx, 238, 286
Campbell, Nelson, 64
Campbell, T. Colin, 8, 17, 64, 96, 173,
    181
cancer, xiv, xv, 8, 9, 27, 44–49, 184,
    185
    meat and, 47, 56
    soy and, 118–19
carbs, junk, 183
carnism, 55
carnivores, 23–24
Carrot Cake, Suzy's, 275–76
cashews:
    Cashew-Hazelnut Milk, 125

Pagie Poo's "Cazzewww" Cream,
    257–58
Ree Ree's Cheese Spread, 255–56
Centers for Disease Control and
    Prevention (CDC), 51, 100, 101
Chatham House, 95, 100
cheese, 7, 50, 76, 82, 96, 139–40
Cheesecake Mousse, Pagie Poo's
    Lemon, 277–78
cheeses, plant-based, 140, 200
    Ree Ree's Cheese Spread, 255–56
Cheese Trap, The (Barnard), 96
"chicken":
    BBQ "Chicken" Sliders with Classic
        Coleslaw, 236–37
    "Chicken" Fajitas, 227–28
    Curried "Chicken" Salad in Lettuce
        Cups, 229
children:
    in the kitchen, 158–59
    lunches for, 143, 149
    nutrition for, 51–54
    vegetables and, 143, 162–63
chili, 147–48, 231, 233
    Suzy's Family Favorite Chili, 230
Chili Sauce, Mom Cameron's, 261–63
China, 81
China Study, The (Campbell), 17, 35,
    96, 181
chocolate:
    Dark Chocolate Lamington Cakes
        with Blackberry Sorbet, 270–73
    Food Forest Organics Coco-Mint
        Slice, 279–81
    Green Chocolate Milk Smoothie, 201
    Pagie Poo's Chocolate Mousse,
        278–79
cholesterol, xvii, 26, 31–33, 38, 173,
    184–85
climate change, xvii–xviii, xix, xxiii,
    12, 17, 61–72, 77, 80, 87, 135, 285
    animal agriculture and, 11, 49–50,
        62, 65–66, 69–71, 81
    Paris Agreement and, 65, 66, 137
    regional effects of, 66–68, 101
Climatic Change, 137
Coconut Cream, Whipped, 274–75

Coconut-Lemon-Blueberry Scones, 211–12
coconut milk, 122, 123
Coleslaw, Classic, BBQ "Chicken" Sliders with, 236–37
Coming Back to Life (Macy), 87
Consumer Reports, 183
Coodle Cups with Dill-icious Mango Sauce, Melissa's, 219–21
corn:
    Corn Salsa, 254
    The King's Shepherd's Pie, 241–43
    Mom Amis's Creamed Corn, 231–32
    Open-Faced Peppers, 239–40
Costner, Kevin, 5
cravings, 184–86, 197
CSA (Community Supported Agriculture), 99, 128, 199

D

D₃, 115
dairy, 7–11, 38, 44, 71, 73, 81–84, 96, 179
    bone health and, 122–23
    cheese, 7, 50, 76, 82, 96, 139–40
    milk, 36, 47, 50, 76, 81–84, 102, 123, 179
dead zones, 75–76
DEEPSEA CHALLENGE Expedition, 69–70
desserts:
    Dark Chocolate Lamington Cakes with Blackberry Sorbet, 270–73
    Food Forest Organics Coco-Mint Slice, 279–81
    Pagie Poo's Lemon Cheesecake Mousse, 277–78
    Pagie Poo's Chocolate Mousse, 278–79
    Saranne's Meringues, 273–74
    Suzy's Carrot Cake, 275–76
    Whipped Coconut Cream, 274–75
DHA, 53, 111–13
diabetes, xiv, xv, 9, 26, 27, 34–38, 173
Dill-icious Mango Sauce, Melissa's Coodle Cups with, 219–21
dinner recipes, 230–52

dips and spreads:
    Aaron's Eggplant Dip, 252–53
    Aaron's Sweet Potato Hummus, 256–57
    Really Great Guacamole, 254–55
    Ree Ree's Cheese Spread, 255–56
doctors, 34–35, 180–81, 184

E

Eating You Alive, 39
E. coli, 100
Eggplant Dip, Aaron's, 252–53
Elliott, Brad and Sandy, 250
endothelial cells, 31–33
energy, eating for, 53
environment, 284, 286–89
    biodiversity, 73–75
    forests, xviii, 11, 72–73
    Green Eater Meter, xxiv, 103–8, 168, 184, 200, 293
    impact of protein foods, 102
    local concerns, 101–3
    oceans, 11, 75–76
    OMD and, 61–89, 154
    plant-based diet and, xxiii–xxiv, 11–13, 61–89, 197
    water usage, xviii, 11, 76–77, 142, 172, 286
    see also animal agriculture; climate change
EPA, 53, 111–13
erectile function, 37–39, 143
Esselstyn, Caldwell, 8, 64, 173
Esselstyn, Rip, 16, 64
essential fatty acids, 53
estrogen, 118
European Public Health Alliance, 100
"eww factor," 179

F

Fajitas, "Chicken," 227–28
Falafel, Fantastic, 222–24
farmers' markets, 99–100, 103, 128, 199
fats, 112, 185
fiber, 49
fish, 47, 53
fish oil supplements, 112

five-second rule, 139–40
flavor, 95–96
Foley, Jonathan, 69
Food Forest Organics, xx, 286
Food Forest Organics Burgers, 238–39
Food Forest Organics Coco-Mint
    Slice, 279–81
food labels, 178–79
food safety, 100–101
food storage containers and utensils,
    294
Ford, Eileen, 3–4
forests, xviii, 11, 72–73
Forks Over Knives, 8–10, 14–15, 17, 20,
    23, 30, 35, 50, 178, 265
Foster, David, 33–34
French Toast, Rose's, 210–11
Freston, Kathy, 16, 137–38, 168, 227
fruits, 32, 51, 98, 127–30, 160, 199
    Breakfast MUSE-li, 205
    in children's lunches, 143
    colors of, 156
    increasing intake of, 153–62
    Jasper's Green Shake, 201–2
    Jasper's Red Shake, 203
    MUSE-li Mix, 204
    shopping for, 128–29, 131–35
    storing, 129–30, 131–35

G

Game Changers, The, 39, 43, 117
Gascoigne, David, 265
genes, xiv, 9
glucose, 52
Gore, Al, 72
government subsidies, 153
grab-and-go foods, 150–51
Green Eater Meter, xxiv, 103–8, 168,
    184, 200, 293
greenhouse gas emissions, 11, 63,
    65–66, 70–72, 106–8, 142, 168
Gregor, Michael, 17, 181, 183
Guacamole, Really Great, 254–55

H

Harvard T. H. Chan School of Public
    Health, 97

Harvard University, 58
Hazelnut, Parsnip, and Pear
    Pithiviers, 268–70
health, 21–60
    goals for, 24–25
    see also specific subjects
heart disease, xiv, xvi, xvii, 8, 9, 27,
    29–34, 46, 184
    erectile dysfunction and, 37–39
    reversal of, 33–34, 59
hemp milk, 122
herbivores, 23–24
herbs, 149–50
hobo dinners, 162
How Not to Die (Greger), 17, 181
Hyman, Mark, 56–57

I

immune system, 31, 48–49
inflammation, 9, 31, 43, 48, 185
ingredients, 109, 200
insulin-like growth factor (IGF), 47
iodine, 114
IQ, 52

J

JAMA, 118
JAMA Internal Medicine, 36
Jicama Salad, 241
Jones, Sarah, 177
*Journal of the Academy of Nutrition
    and Dietetics,* 40
*Journal of the American College of
    Cardiology,* 97
*Journal of the American College of
    Nutrition,* 37
*Journal of the American Osteopathic
    Association,* 172
Joy, Melanie, 55, 56
junk carbs, 183

K

Kahler, Taibi, 64
kale:
    Jasper's Green Shake, 201–2
    Rio's Marinated Kale Salad, 218–19
Kateman, Brian, 103

Katz, David, 56, 57, 93, 135, 136
King, Jeff, 14, 17, 241
kitchen pantry, 109, 127, 181–82, 295–300
knife, 146–47
Krautwich, Davien's Superb, 221–22

L

Lasagna, Brad and Sandy's Sun-Dried Tomato and Asparagus, 250–52
lemon:
    Lemon-Blueberry-Coconut Scones, 211–12
    Pagie Poo's Lemon Cheesecake Mousse, 277–78
lentils:
    Food Forest Organics Burgers, 238–39
    The King's Shepherd's Pie, 241–43
life expectancy, xv, 9, 26, 50, 57–60, 172–73
Lifestyle Heart Trial, 33
linoleic acid (LA), 53
Littlefield, Davien, 5, 21–22, 41–42, 221
Livestock—Climate Change's Forgotten Sector: Global Public Opinion on Meat and Dairy Consumption, 95
Loma Linda University, 52, 184
lunches:
    for children, 143, 149
    recipes for, 215–29

M

Macy, Joanna, 87
Manaus Conference on Global Sustainability, 72
Mango Sauce, Dill-icious, Melissa's Coodle Cups with, 219–21
mason jars, 126
Mayo Clinic, 172
McCaw, Craig, 64
McDonald's, xvi, 81, 82
McDougall, John, 64, 173, 180
McDougall, Mary, 64
meal planning, 186, 187–95

meat, meat-based diet, xvii–xviii, xxiii, 7–11, 16, 19, 22–24, 32, 38, 42–44
    cancer and, 47, 56
    cutting down on, 147
    demand for, 81–85
    diabetes and, 36
    "four Ns" of, 55–57
    health and, 25–28, 30, 31, 40
    price of, 98–99, 101, 199–200
    treating like cake, 178
    see also animal agriculture; beef
meat analogues, 39, 57, 84, 141
Medical Journal of Australia, 112
Mejia, Maximino Alfredo, xxiv, 104, 200
menus:
    14-day OMD All-In plan, 187–95
    special event, 266–73
Merchants of Doubt, 285
Meringues, Saranne's, 273–74
metric conversions, 313
Mexican fiesta, 156
microbiome, 48
milk, 36, 47, 50, 76, 81–84, 102, 123, 179
milks, plant-based, 83–84, 121–25
    making your own, 125, 214–15
miso, 114
Moby, 16
muscle mass, 42–43
MUSE-li, 205
MUSE-li Mix, 204
MUSE School, xi, xii, xx, xxiv, 7–8, 13–19, 50–51, 74, 89, 104–5, 137–38, 144, 175, 229, 241, 286
MUSE Talks, 16
MUSE-Y Joes, 225–26

N

Nachum, Zoe, 160–61
NASA, 71
National Geographic, 70
Nature, 27
NGOs, 12, 62, 64, 74, 285, 288
niacin, 153
NPR, 103

Nurses' Health Study, 32
nutrition, 110–15
  for children, 51–54
nutritional yeast ("nooch"), 152–53
Nutrition Reviews, 40
nuts, 97, 185
  Ben's Apple-Walnut "Mouffins,"
    213–14
  MUSE-li Mix, 204
  nut butters, 145–46, 185
  Ree Ree's Raw Vegan Taco Nut
    "Meat," 226–27

O

oats:
  MUSE-li Mix, 204
  Oatmeal with Roasted Peaches,
    207–8
obesity, 40–41
oceans, 11, 75–76
Okra and Tomatoes, Scooter's,
  235–36
olive oil, 109
OMD (One Meal a Day), xi–xii,
    xxi–xxv, 19–20, 86, 88, 135–36,
    137–70, 174, 179–80, 287–89
  All-In, *see* All-In
  birth of, 13–19
  brain trust, xxiv, 17, 20, 23, 50–51,
    173
  buddy for, 139
  environmental benefits of, 61–89,
    154
  flower diagram, 28, 62–63, 68, 73,
    88, 285
  14-day transition plan for, 164–67
  14-day transition plan shopping
    list, 301–4
  gentle start, 147–67
  Green Eater Meter, xxiv, 103–8,
    168, 184, 200, 293
  health benefits of, 21–60
  master pantry list, 295–300
  motivation factors in, 95–103
  pledge, 89
  preparation for, 93–136
  public health and, 49–50

recipes for, *see* recipes
stepping up, 168–69
omega-3 fatty acids, 53, 111–13
Oppenlander, Richard, 64
Ornish, Dean, 33–34, 51, 59–60, 64,
    115, 118, 123, 173, 180, 181, 184

P

Pampanin, Melissa, 219–20
Pancakes with Mixed Berry Syrup,
    208–9
pancreatitis, 35
pantry, 109, 127, 181–82, 295–300
Paris Agreement, 65, 66, 137
Parsnip, Hazelnut, and Pear
    Pithiviers, 268–70
pasta, 158
  Brad and Sandy's Sun-Dried
    Tomato and Asparagus Lasagna,
    250–52
  Quinn's Pesto, 260
  Spaghetti Bolognese, 246–47
Patel, Raj, 82
Peaches, Roasted, Oatmeal with, 207–8
peanut butter and jelly, 145
Peanut Sauce, Jasper's, 259
pea protein milk, 121, 122, 125
Pear, Parsnip, and Hazelnut
    Pithiviers, 268–70
pepper, 109
Peppers, Open-Faced, 239–40
Pesto, Quinn's, 260
pizza, 140, 158
plant-based eating, 283–89
  environment and, xxiii–xxiv,
    11–13, 61–89, 197
  health benefits of, xxiii–xxiv, 8–11,
    24, 26–29, 32–33, 35–37, 46, 57
  IQ and, 52
  longevity and, 9, 50, 57–60
  public health and, 49–50
  use of term, 180, 195–96
  weight loss and, 40
Plant Power Task Force, xx, 286
plastic, 130, 131
Pollan, Michael, xxiii
polyphenols, 32–33

Pooley, Eric, 64
pressure cookers, 231, 233–35
price, 98–99
    of meat, 98–99, 101, 199–200
protein, 6, 30, 42–44
    amino acids in, 52, 117
    animal, xv, xvi, 16, 30
    environmental impact of foods,
        102
    plant sources of, 117–18
    progression, 142–43
    requirements for, 115–17

Q
quesadillas, 162
quinoa:
    Josa's Garlicky Quinoa Salad with
        Spring Vegetables, 248–49
    Open-Faced Peppers, 239–40

R
recipes, xxiv, 199–281
    baked goods and desserts, 273–81
    breakfast, 201–14
    dinner sides and main dishes,
        230–52
    lunch, 215–29
    snacks, spreads, and dips, 252–65
Red Carpet Green Dress, xx, 286
Reddy, Patsy, 199, 265–66
Reynolds, Kevin, 5
rice, 183–84, 234
    Food Forest Organics Burgers,
        238–39
Robards, Sam, 5, 6, 179
Robbins, John, 64
Robbins, Mel, 139–40
Roll, Rich, 16
Ronnen, Tal, 16, 141–42

S
safety, food, 100–101
salad dressings:
    Aaron's Ranch Dressing,
        264–65
    Pagie Poo's Delicious Salad
        Dressing, 263–64

salads, 155–56, 161
    Curried "Chicken" Salad in Lettuce
        Cups, 229
    Jicama Salad, 241
    Josa's Garlicky Quinoa Salad with
        Spring Vegetables, 248–49
    Rio's Marinated Kale Salad, 218–19
Salsa, Corn, 254
salt, 109
sauces:
    Jasper's Peanut Sauce, 259
    Mom Cameron's Chili Sauce, 261–63
    Quinn's Pesto, 260
schools, lunch options at, 149, 288
Science, 75
Scones, Lemon-Blueberry-Coconut,
    211–12
sea levels, 71–72
Seventh-day Adventists, 36, 110, 184
sex, 37–39
Shepherd's Pie, The King's, 241–43
Shiva, Vandana, 85, 286
slow cookers, 148–49, 231
smoking, 284–85
smoothies and shakes:
    Green Chocolate Milk Smoothie,
        201
    Jasper's Green Shake, 201–2
    Jasper's Red Shake, 203
Soltani, Atossa, 72
soups, 161
    Heirloom Tomato Consommé,
        266–67
    Saranne's Roasted "Cream" of
        Tomato Soup, 217–18
    Spinach-Sweet Potato Soup, 215–16
soy, 118–19
    soy milk, 122, 124
    tempeh, 119–21
    tofu, see tofu
Spaghetti Bolognese, 246–47
Spielberg, Steven, 5
spinach:
    Green Chocolate Milk Smoothie, 201
    Jasper's Green Shake, 201–2
    Spinach-Sweet Potato Soup, 215–16
Spitz, Aaron, 39

spreads, *see* dips and spreads
spring rolls, 159
Cheri and Charlie's Spring Rolls,
243–45
sweet potatoes:
Aaron's Sweet Potato Hummus,
256–57
Spinach-Sweet Potato Soup, 215–16

T
takeout foods, 141
telomeres and telomerase, xiv–xv, 9,
59, 60
tempeh, 119–21
Theiss, Brian, 29–31
TMAO (trimethylamine-N-oxide),
32–33
tofu, 119–20
Brad and Sandy's Sun-Dried
Tomato and Asparagus Lasagna,
250–52
Scrambled Tofu, 205–6
tomatoes, 235
Brad and Sandy's Sun-Dried
Tomato and Asparagus Lasagna,
250–52
Heirloom Tomato Consommé,
266–67
Mom Cameron's Chili Sauce,
261–63
Saranne's Roasted "Cream" of
Tomato Soup, 217–18
Scooter's Okra and Tomatoes,
235–36
Spaghetti Bolognese, 246–47
Suzy's Family Favorite Chili, 230
Totorici, Elle, 175–76
Tufts University, 52
Tyson Foods, 84

U
Ulithi, 49, 69–70, 72
umami, 152
United Nations Food and Agriculture
Organization, 71
University of Oxford, 77

V
Veganist (Freston), 16, 227
vegans, 21, 23, 36, 40–42, 55, 56, 117,
180, 195–98, 285
vegetables, 32, 51, 98, 99, 109, 127–30,
199
children and, 143, 162–63
colors of, 156
increasing intake of, 153–62
layering on, 156
pickled, 222
preparing, 161, 182
shopping for, 128–29, 131–35
storing, 129–30, 131–35
veggie tray, 155–56
vegetarians, 36, 37, 40–41, 56, 65, 117,
172, 180, 283, 285
Verdient Foods, 286
vinegars, 109
vitamin B_{12}, 110–11
vitamin D_3, 115
Vogel, Robert, xvi

W
Walmart, 284
walnuts:
Ben's Apple-Walnut "Mouffins,"
213–14
MUSE-li Mix, 204
Ree Ree's Raw Vegan Taco Nut
"Meat," 226–27
Washor, Elliot, 8
water usage, xviii, 11, 76–77, 142, 172,
286
weight loss, 40–42
Wilks, James, 39
wolves, 74
World Health Organization (WHO),
47, 56
World Meteorological Organization,
71
World Resources Institute,
154

Y
yogurt, plant-based, 234–35

About the Author

A noted environmental advocate, actor, and mother of five, Suzy Amis Cameron is committed to the principles of sustainability in all aspects of our lives, with emphasis on plant-based solutions to address climate change. Currently, she is a founder of Plant Power Task Force, focused on showing the impact of animal agriculture on climate change and the environment, with her husband James Cameron. In 2005 she founded MUSE School with her sister Rebecca Amis. MUSE recently became the first school in the country to be 100 percent solar powered, zero waste, and with a 100 percent organic, plant-based lunch program. Additionally, she is a founder of Verdient, Cameron Family Farms, and Food Forest Organics, all plant-based initiatives, and Red Carpet Green Dress, showcasing socially and environmentally responsible fashions. Suzy has executive produced documentaries and serves on several non-profit boards. As an actor she was featured in more than twenty-five films, including *The Usual Suspects* and *Titanic*.